Healthy Teeth

=

Healthy Life

Why Oral Care is Vital to Wellness

Anthony Mikalauskas

Authors note:

There are many different therapies, systems, procedures and protocols other than what may be outlined here. I am not a dentist, just someone who has a passion for human life, the body we reside in now, quality of life, staying healthy through nutrition and supplements, and helping others as much as possible. I studied a more holistic approach to life and nutrition in the Philippines for 2 years, learning how to help people with different types of deficiencies in an all-natural way. Trying to find supplements with the best efficacy and ability to help with different diseases, ailments, and disorders.

There are many more options available besides the natural ones I have mentioned in this book. Please consult your doctor who knows your medical history before making any changes to any medications or lifestyles.

Anyone who has questions about nutrition or all natural systems are free to email or text me, and if I can help I will gladly give you all the information I have.

4mulanutrition@gmail.com

312.476.9408

INTRODUCTION

After being in the fitness and nutrition industry for twenty plus years, I have always been interested in two things....

1. *HELPING*

   PEOPLE

   And....

2. *THE MARVEL*

   OF THE

   HUMAN

   BODY

A very intelligent and close mentor of mine always told me that if you make helping people your priority, as a byproduct you will receive everything you would want and need to make sure you can maintain the ability to continue helping people in the future as well as maintaining a good life for yourself. As far as the marvel of the human body, what this meant to me in the past was the muscular and skeletal system. How exercise strengthened the heart and blood circulation, how the muscle could speed up your metabolism, and the different brain chemicals released while working out and after could alter your mood and attitude in a way not even medications could. As time went by, I started to realize how important a role *nutrition* played and how much you could manipulate your size, strength, and even personality based on nutrition.

As I trained individuals with diabetes, cancer, heart disease, hip and knee replacements, and many other issues some of us are not even aware of, I eventually took a step back and noticed that it was such a problem in so many different people and personalities from various walks of life. Some of the things that I was curious about was how so many different people could all have the same problems in life. For example, growing up, I was always told not to smoke because you would most certainly get cancer and die. Now I have never smoked or had cancer, but I have trained many people who had cancer and never smoked or even had an alcoholic beverage in their lives. Diabetes was yet another mind boggling condition I could not wrap my head around. So many doctors I spoke with would tell me that it's just what happens once you start getting older. However, the more people I trained, the more I started to see that cancer, diabetes, and all the others did NOT seem to discriminate with age, sex, nationality, or religion. I have trained a 14 year old that had terminal cancer, and I have watched a 62 year old man who NEVER smoked a day in his life, ran marathons and would race me up the stairs at the gym when I was 24 years old pass away from pancreatic cancer. How do you explain those 2 people or blame one or two different substances? I had a home client that would exercise with his daughter while I trained him because she was at risk for diabetes. Not to mention the fact that we are living in a country that promotes milk and other dairy products in a large majority of our foods so that we can strengthen our bones with calcium and vitamin D. So how do you explain the fact that we have so many bone fractures in the USA while some countries that DO NOT promote milk in the daily diet have much less? Or the fact that when an elderly person "falls down and breaks a hip", the truth is that they did the opposite and fell after the hip just happened to break?

This drove me for many years to read, watch, and learn the body, as well as how to fix certain muscle imbalances and injuries, and put a strong emphasis on nutrition. The ability to change your body based on what you eat has since been such a phenomenon to me. I later found out that the right amount of certain amino acids, proteins, and removal of certain poisonous foods such as sugar can adjust your endocrine system. The endocrine system can cause havoc if there is a problem. Things such as Thyroid issues that so many people suffer from can be reversed by eating the correct foods.

Then after a few years, I began to question, why did some people brush their teeth on a regular basis and still get cavities, while others rarely brushed and seemed to have strong teeth?

I then began to read, study, and watch as much as I could about teeth, the oral microbiome, the amount of good and bad bacteria that is in your mouth, and the problems that can occur if there is an imbalance. I also studied the types of probiotics you can use to help eliminate certain problems such as gingivitis, thrush, canker sores, cavities and obviously a list of issues we can have. The fact that we can find specific bacteria that can help with each problem individually shows that it can also be avoided, but the question is how?

The other thing I started to wonder was, if everything starts with our mouths and what we put inside of it, could we also get sick by not taking good care of our teeth and gums? Or was our teeth solely for chewing food and looking pretty with a white smile? If our mouths are the first thing we take care of in the morning and the last thing we take care of at night, oral hygiene must mean more than just our physical appearance and a cute smile. It is also something to ponder on as to why there has not been an innovative brushing system until now. The importance of having a wellness system such as vitamins and supplements for our body is essential to our lives. How much more should it be considered to have a wellness system for the very thing that EVERYTHING we take into our bodies passes through.

After further research, there are a large number of diseases that can start with poor oral hygiene.

1. **DIABETES**- 95% of people with diabetes will experience some form of gum disease.

2. LEUKEMIA- Gingivitis can be an early symptom of leukemia.

3. HEART DISEASE

These are just a few of the diseases that can start with poor oral hygiene. This is not including the number of poisons we use to brush our teeth, carcinogens we use to rinse our mouths with, and the toxins we fill our bodies with throughout the day. We will go over some of the most dangerous ones that can be avoided so that we not only keep our teeth white and happy with a healthy smile, but also live a longer healthier life.

We will learn the history of the toothbrush as well as toothpaste so that we can see what was used hundreds of years ago, why it worked or didn't work, and what we have done to make improvements with the tools we use to keep our smile pretty and stay alive in the process. What kind of toxins are being used in the toothpaste and mouthwash, and what are the reasons they are using these poisons in our mouths? We will learn how we can get the proper bacteria into places such as under the tooth so as to fight off possible infections or bad bacteria, as well as some of the damages and health concerns that come with listening to some of the popular mainstream lies that are being told, and how we can avoid some of them if possible. When it comes to anything medical, be it doctors with nutrition and exercise or dentists with oral hygiene, there are always things that seem like you need to have a translator just to know how to be healthy. In this book, I am hoping I can explain things so we can all easily understand them after you are finished. This is a problem I used to have many years ago when it came to nutrition and trying to understand what nutrients mix better with others. Now we are learning not just how important oral hygiene is, but also the many ways it can benefit our lives and wellbeing for decades to come.

Trust me when I tell you that you will not only thank us because you look better, but you will also feel better and healthier. Your friends and family will most likely also thank us for the change in you. Now let's get started on your journey to start living the healthiest way possible, and transform you into the best possible you that there is through a few oral wellness options that nobody seems to be telling us.

Table of contents

Chapter 1:

Does my life depend on my teeth?

We all know everyone wants white teeth as the result of consistent brushing. Great smelling breath is obviously just as important. But what if you found out that neglecting your teeth, or caring for your mouth as a whole could be detrimental to your health? What if you found out that it could cause things such as diabetes, heart disease, rheumatoid arthritis, or on a severe stretch, possible death? Would this start making you a little more likely to brush those teeth? Here, we will take a look at how neglecting to brush your teeth can cause some of the most life threatening and debilitating diseases we know of. We will look at the process of how your teeth start deteriorating which will lead to so many other problems, in some cases being wheelchair-bound.

ROOT CANALS

Root canals have been such a basic part of life in the dental industry as of the 1980s and 90s. The history goes much further - back to the late 1800s and early 1900s, but the really important dates would be *1943* when The American Association of Endodontics was established to facilitate professional practice in this specialty, and the *1950s* when research established that natural teeth needing root canals do not cause systemic health problems, which in essence told everyone that this was an extremely safe procedure to have done. Then in the *1990s,* Endodontic root canal treatments received an upgrade due to improved imaging techniques, the advent of rotary nickel-titanium files to clean canals, and use of new irrigating solutions.

The history and almost anything having to do with root canals is definitely boring if that's what you were thinking. It's the part where it can have side effects up to and including death that becomes a much more interesting side topic to be discussed.

Naturally we have millions, sometimes even billions of bacteria in our mouths.

Most bacteria that are involved in tooth infections were believed to be aerobic. What this means is that the bacteria would need oxygen to survive. We all know what would happen if we were deprived of oxygen; we would not live very long at all. Well, this is what was assumed for the infection causing bacteria within your mouth. So, it was assumed that when the root canal filling was in place it would eliminate the oxygen, and the bacteria would not be able to survive. If this was the case, then it would make the procedure as safe as they stated many years ago. For many years however, Dr. Price and dozens of scientists on staff, as well as other dentists up until this day have been running extensive tests to understand why so many people would have severe health problems after getting their root canal done.

In the early 1900s Dr. Price began to treat a woman who had been confined to a wheelchair for 6 years because of severe arthritis. Dr. Price, having been working with root canal infections, asked the woman if he could pull the tooth despite there not being any visible signs of infection. After extracting the tooth, the patient left and Dr Price decided to try a few tests he had heard of in the past. He took the root canal-filled tooth and embedded it under the skin of a rabbit. It only took 2 days before the rabbit had developed the same crippling disease the patient was suffering from, and in 10 days the rabbit died of the infection.

Afterwards, Dr Price scheduled a follow-up visit with the woman to see how she was feeling and to also explain his findings. To his surprise, the woman had made a successful recovery and not only was NOT in a wheelchair any longer, but she was able to walk on her own without even a cane to support her. She was even able to do fine needle work once again since her hand was now so steady. Naturally this sparked his interest in continuing the same types of studies in thousands of patients over the years. In almost every instance the test subject would develop the same disease or one very similar. These infections in the test subjects were so devastating that most animals died within 12 days after infection. My next question was, what if you embedded a healthy tooth or cells of some sort, would that give the same effect on the test subject? Dr Price wanted to find out if maybe it was just the tooth being put in the animal that was the cause of the problem. He embedded a healthy tooth, as well as different healthy cells into the rabbits and there was no negative response. The worst thing that happened was the rabbit's immune system sometimes pushed it out to get rid of the foreign object. It turns out that the bacteria they assumed would die with no air did NOT die. It turns out this bacterium is an extremely strong type of beast, and is known as polymorphic. What this means is that it can mutate and change form. During this mutation they would become smaller in size and number, and this would lead the normal person to assume that if the monster (Bad Bacteria) was smaller and there were less of them, then the damage they would cause should be minimal. These smaller monster beasts (Bad Bacteria) now can live without oxygen and at the same time become extremely poisonous or venomous, aggressively interfering with the immune system of the person. So basically, the monster

(Bad Bacteria) is stronger and has intent to hurt, in a manner of speaking. It will leak into the bloodstream and go on a mission looking for anything, including your organs to settle in and cause havoc.

If we can find a really good holistic dentist to give us advice on how we should proceed with infected teeth, we should do that. They will usually give much more natural; sound advice than the average dentist who will just recommend whatever the ADA is pushing them to do. Or we can eliminate these things from happening all together and start taking great care of your teeth, so that this is not a future worry of yours. I personally would brush twice a day with the proper fluoride free toothpaste (reasons covered later) and floss over bacteria that can cause me to have some of the worst diseases I know of. I think this is a great reason why we should brush our teeth and take care of our mouths.

GINGIVITIS

Gingivitis is a non-destructive disease that causes inflammation of the gums. The most common form of gingivitis, and the most common form of periodontal disease overall, is in response to bacterial biofilms attached to tooth surfaces, termed plaque-induced gingivitis. In case you are not aware, the removal of *PLAQUE* is the first step in avoiding all these nasty things. Plaque is what we remove when we brush our teeth in the morning after waking up, and before we go to bed at night.

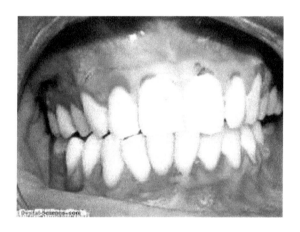

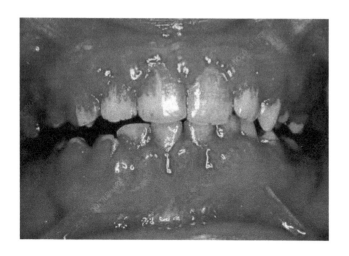

This is a much more severe case of gingivitis obviously. It is highly suggested that you see a dentist well before reaching this point. Typically, after being diagnosed with gingivitis such as this, a surgical procedure will have to take place to remove the gums from the teeth. After the gums have been removed, the dentist will begin to scrape the tartar from the teeth before reattaching the gums. Or we can just make sure that we consistently brush our teeth twice a day, preferably with a system such as Fresh mouth club where you have a new brush every month, fluoride free toothpaste, alcohol free mouthwash, and of course dental floss. I think that would be much more enjoyable than the dentist pulling my gums from my teeth to scrape them.

HALITOSIS (BAD BREATH)

Halitosis, commonly known as bad breath, is a symptom in which a noticeably unpleasant odor is present on the breath. It can result in anxiety among those affected. It is also associated with depression and symptoms of obsessive-compulsive disorder. I can imagine that dragon breath would make someone a little anxious, perhaps even make them feel depressed at times, especially if you could smell your own breath. Most people would have these feelings if they don't know what the cause of your bad breath is or even worse, how to get rid of it.

When you don't brush properly, or often enough, bacteria can form in your mouth, and it's one of the primary causes of bad breath. This bacteria feeds on the food particles left behind on your teeth and gums and produces waste products which release foul odors. If you have braces, you should take extra care to remove food particles from your mouth in order to avoid bad breath. Personally, the thought of bacteria in my mouth is enough of a wake-up call to brush my teeth on a regular basis. The idea of that same bacteria feeding off the food particles that are left between my teeth and leaving fecal matter (POOP) after they have full bellies behind in my mouth and making it smell..... well..... like POOP, is more than enough incentive to brush at least twice a day and floss in the middle to get rid of those food particles in the first place so I can avoid this from happening all together.

Chapter 2:

Importance of Oral Microbiome

According to Wikipedia the word microbiome was first used by J.L. Mohr in 1952 in *The Scientific Monthly* to imply that the microorganisms that were found in a specific environment. It was defined in 1988 by Whipps et al. as "a characteristic microbial community occupying a reasonably well-defined habitat which has distinct physio-chemical properties. Thus, the term not only refers to the microorganisms involved, but also encompasses their theater of activity".

To use a more simplified approach, we will use the military as an example. If there was a foreign threat within our country and we were all in danger of mass injuries, sicknesses and even death, the **microbiome** would represent our **Military,** the divisions that are involved, and what the attack plans would be. So our microbiome is similar to saying "we are sending the marines to eliminate the violent threat, the Army will keep peace on the streets, and the air force will continue to fly through as backup to wipe out any enemy (bad bacteria) left standing. The meaning behind this is that the threat and the protection are both military soldiers. It's only a matter of who the good guys and the bad guys are, and who is more prepared for battle.

Now despite what you may hear from our friends on the television that speak about fluoride toothpaste or mouthwash and how successful they are at killing ALL the bacteria in your mouth, it is important to understand that we have over 800 different types of bacteria in our mouth, many of which are fighting for you and your **increased** health. That being said, It is NOT in your best interest to kill all of the germs in your mouth. In fact, some of the germs living in your oral cavity are essential for healthy living.

So why is it that we continue to use on our teeth, products that are essentially laced with different types of poison that studies have shown can make our teeth yellow, and go as far as lowering children's I.Q? Well, this widespread destruction of our oral microbiome can be blamed in part on our dentists who are the ones who refer to such products to help keep our mouths in good health. In their defense, Dentists are in no way trained in any school, be it a university or a specialty dental school, to treat the oral microbiome, which would lead to the conclusion that they are not taught how to nourish, rebuild, or protect the oral microbiome.

Like a doctor, the approach a dentist takes is typically very reactive as opposed to proactive. Which means that when there is a problem, such as a cavity, gingivitis, or gum disease, they react to the situation by performing the known procedure. This however is vastly different from the proactive approach of changing whatever the habit was that caused the problem in the first place. Instead, some of the dentist's views of "wellness" include strictly focusing on the health and superficial condition of their client's teeth, whom they encourage to use different types of teeth whitening products, and all the while not realizing that this could potentially disrupt the capabilities of their client's microbiomes, which, in turn, could result in severe, negative ramifications for their patient's overall state of health.

To achieve an optimal state of oral and physical health, instead of killing **ALL** the mouth's bacteria with alcoholic mouthwash, one must focus on balancing the mouth's diverse microbial ecology. The question would be how can this be done? I think first we should try to get a brief understanding as to what the microbiome is, and how we can either help or hinder it throughout our day.

As stated earlier, there are over 800 different bacteria forming your oral microbiome. For the sake of keeping this simple and somewhat easy to understand, we will talk about how these fall into one of 3 categories.

- **Symbiotic**

- **Commensal** · **Pathogenic**

Symbiotic means having a close, cooperative, or interdependent relationship. A good example of this is how most people have a symbiotic type relationship with their dog.

Commensal (of an animal, plant, fungus, etc.) living with, on, or in another, without injury to either. We can think of this as being the unbiased party of the group. This is the person who does not vote in the election, they just go about their day as best as possible.

Pathogenic is any small organism, such as a virus or a bacterium that can cause disease. I think it is safe to say that these are the bad guys.

Now all things considered, if you were just told this, it would seem like it's a pretty fair game. You have the good guys on one side, the bad guys on the other, and an audience that watches as non-biased fans. Where the problem lies is that just as human beings like to win -even if we are not on a specific side- so do the commensal(unbiased) bacteria. With this being said, the problem lies when the bad bacteria start to gain in numbers; there is a good chance they could possibly bully the commensal bacteria to pick a specific side and actually join the fight.

Imagine starting off your morning, you wake, stroll into the bathroom where you begin your daily process of caring for your teeth. After brushing (hopefully with Fluoride free toothpaste) and rinsing out your mouth, you feel the caring for your teeth part is over. It's really just begun for the bacteria inside, good or bad, and they are now getting to work. Before continuing, let's keep in mind that just as there are good and bad bacteria, there are good and bad plaque.

The first thing that would take place is our saliva interacting with the surface of our enamel to form the **PELLICLE**. The pellicle is a protective protein which starts to form almost immediately after we are finished brushing them. Aerobic (oxygen loving/good) bacteria will begin to attach to it. This will create a thin and *NOT* sticky layer of *good* plaque/biofilm. The good bacteria(symbiotic) and neutral (commensal) tend to be aerobic, which means they thrive on oxygen.

Now as we start our day and have our morning coffee, possibly a pastry of some sort, and maybe some eggs for breakfast, this marks the start of the daily war inside of your mouth that we are all unaware of. Now is when there are other microbes beginning to attach to the biofilm. Many of these microbes produce a *sticky* enzyme which thickens the biofilm and allows more diverse species to join the colony. So sticky **plaque**/biofilm is bad, and NOT sticky is generally good or neutral. The reason for this is that as the plaque/biofilm begins to thicken and become stickier, there is a decline in the amount of oxygen that can enter the biofilm. Bear in mind that GOOD bacteria thrive on oxygen, and BAD bacteria want extraordinarily little oxygen. The process of the biofilm going from aerobic to anaerobic is where the creation of what we know as **PLAQUE** begins to take place. This is the plaque that we all know to be bad, which has a whitish color and is generally sticky, thus making it harder to leave.

This anaerobic/lower oxygen environment creates an ideal ecosystem for PATHOGENIC (disease causing) bacteria to start populating stronger and colonizing the biofilm. If this is allowed to continue, then the biofilm will no doubt continue to thicken and strangle the available oxygen more and more until there is a rapid microbial balance shift. This is where the good bacteria meant to protect and heal are no longer in control due to the low oxygenated environment.

Not only is this where the pathogens/bad bacteria begin to take over and run things due to the lower oxygenated environment - remember when we discussed the neutral (commensal) bacteria and their likeliness of choosing to side with whatever team is winning? Maybe the lack of oxygen makes them brain dead, but this is where they fall in place and start to follow orders from the pathogens. So now, the pathogens/BAD bacteria have just increased their army and colonies exponentially. If this is allowed to continue and we let it get out of hand, it then takes us to what we know as TARTAR buildup.

TARTAR/CALCULUS- Tartar is a form of hardened dental plaque. It is caused by precipitation of minerals from saliva and gingival crevicular fluid in plaque on the teeth.

When we get to the level of heavy tartar buildup, it means that these vicious microbes have built a hardened fortress of calcified plaque in their colonies to protect them while they do their dirty work. The question here would be,

what exactly does their dirty work entail?

Well once these colonies are fully grown and dominated by

disease-causing microbes, they will now engage in the work of trying to steal as many minerals from you as possible, such as calcium and phosphorus. These minerals are in your saliva, and they are needed to remineralize your teeth. So our goal would be to avoid any of this from taking place now that we are aware of what starts to happen after we brush our teeth. We want to do all that we can to enrich the biofilm with oxygen and stay thin so we can be sure to protect our teeth throughout the day.

How to keep the good guys strong

There are a few things that we can focus on to make sure that we don't ever get to the point of our symbiotic oral flora (THE GOOD GUYS) being overthrown by the violent, teeth damaging pathogenic bad bacteria.

1.   Making sure that we have an abundance of fat-soluble vitamins in our diet. Either through food or supplementation this can somewhat easily be accomplished. Vitamins D, E, and K2 are all very important.

Vitamin D can be found in salmon, tuna, egg yolks, and mushrooms.

Studies have shown that a large portion of the world population is very low on Vitamin D3. This can be helped with the proper supplementation.

Vitamin E can be found in several foods such as peanuts, advocado, almonds, lobster, and many other nuts. According to healthline some of the problems that can occur when deficient in Vitamin E are difficulty with walking or coordination, muscle pain or weakness, visual disturbances, and general unwellness.

Vitamin K2 can be found in eggs, pepperoni, sour cream, and most types of chicken.

2.   Having plenty of vitamins B and C in our diet as well as high amounts of minerals are extremely important factors for our oral health.

Vitamin B is a little more involved, being that there are 8 different types of B vitamins. Going through all of them is not of great importance currently. The main thing you need to keep in mind is that B12 is the only one that your body can hold onto for a long period of time, which means you will need to constantly keep replacing them from food sources throughout the day. There are many foods that contain B vitamins. Some good sources include Salmon,

Leafy greens, organ meats, Eggs, milk and beef.

3.   Staying away from sugar in all forms is especially important, as I'm sure we are all aware of.

I'm sure at this point you must be wondering why it seems to be that there is so much involved with nutrition and bad habits when it comes to our teeth and oral health. Most people assume that teeth are just types of bones, and as long as we don't do anything physically damaging and stay away from sweets we can maintain them forever. Well if that were true, then there would not be millions of individuals around the world who have been brushing twice a day with their fluoride toothpaste, rinsing their mouths with mouthwash, and getting cleanings twice a year wondering why they are still getting cavities.

Are Teeth Alive?

A study done by Dr. Steinman found that not only are our teeth alive, but they also have fluid running through them which is referred to as "dentinal fluid flow". This is part of the blood circulation that goes in and out of each of our teeth. What he found out about the dentinal fluid flow was that if it flows from the inside of the tooth and then outward, the teeth are almost impossible to decay. It would be like the bad bacteria having to swim upstream during a hurricane before even attempting to start doing damage. However, when the fluid flows from the outer surface of the tooth and towards the inner portion, then decay can set in pretty easily. Almost as if the guards fell asleep at the gate leaving it wide open for those nasty bad bacteria to walk right in.

To try and make this as simplistic as possible, what causes the dentinal fluid to flow in one direction as opposed to the other is the balance of the mineral *phosphorus* in our blood. This is why diet and nutrition are so important in whether we experience resistance to decay or are prone to it.

So basically, what we need to know is exactly what causes low blood phosphorus levels so we can avoid this. One thing to keep in mind is that if we have certain pre-existing conditions, it may cause some problems, such as your phosphorus level going down if you have high cholesterol, glucose, or calcium. Another problem is the way our food has been grown for close to the last 100 years it has been deficient in many of the trace minerals we need.

Therefore, it is imperative to enrich our diets with the proper amounts of vitamins and minerals. This can also become more difficult when a large amount of the population has digestion issues due to an unhealthy microbiome. Some of the foods we can make sure that we start taking in are.....

More healthy fats:

Dr. Price was a dentist that traveled the world to study people that did not start taking in the western diet of poisons. What he found was nothing short of amazing. After examining 100 skulls he found only 1 cavity. The reason he came to this conclusion was that other cultures eat 4 times more minerals and 10 times more fats than people living in industrial communities. Consuming high quality fats helps us get the minerals our teeth require. This will help in digesting the fat-soluble vitamins and strengthen your teeth as well as many other parts of the body.

Quality foods are especially important, and organic is probably the best source of animal products. For example, the amount of K2 in animal products drops significantly when the animal is not raised on green grass. Some of the other foods are....

Eggs

Organ meats of cattle

Pastured chicken

Wild caught fish

Dairy products

Bone broth

Sauerkraut.

ProBiotics

As of mid-2020, 8 randomized, controlled trials on oral probiotics for dental caries have been completed. 75% of these studies found that the use of dental probiotics reduced cavities, with the oral microbiome being one of the most complex and diverse, harboring hundreds of species. The way all these species distribute is determined by a number of factors.

1.   Types of surfaces available: Remember, there are 2 types of surfaces available for colonization in the oral cavity; hard and soft. The presence of hard, non-shedding surfaces is a unique feature of the mouth as tooth surfaces (and dentures) allow the development of permanent communities that will produce their own subdivisions unless disrupted by regular oral hygiene. On the other hand, soft mucosal surfaces promote constant community turnover due to epithelial cell shedding. Both types of surfaces are constantly bathed by saliva.

2. **Oxygen availability:** When we keep our teeth healthy with good oral hygiene, we keep it highly oxygenated. As we talked about earlier, this is the perfect environment for the good bacteria to thrive in and keep the vicious bad bacteria away. As our oral

hygiene is neglected, so is the level of oxygen, which allows these bad bacteria to multiply.

3.   Exposure to nutrients from diet: We have learned that what we eat has a great deal to do with our oral microbiome and if the dentinal flow will be beneficial to protecting our teeth and gums, or will open the door for the attack on our teeth from the bad guys.

So what happens if we don't know exactly what kind of trace minerals we might need, or do not have access to some of the foods that are necessary? Maybe, as stated earlier, we have a health condition that makes it even more difficult to keep up with the proper balance of nutrients. What can we do to help keep our mouth healthy and smiles happy?

Probiotics taken orally can help support your oral health.
They are a type of living organism, and the supplements are generally a combination of various yeasts and bacteria. Bifidobacterium and Lactobacillus are the most common probiotic groups, and there are multiple strains in each of these.

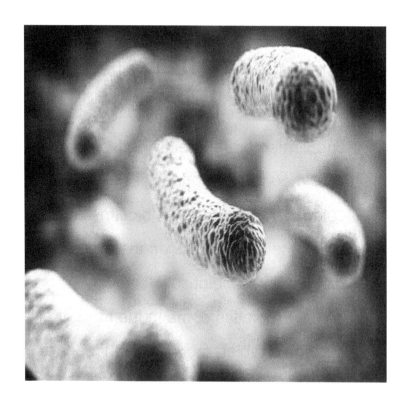

There are microorganism colonies
living in your mouth, and most of these
bacteria are not bad. Those classified
as probiotics are beneficial to your
dental health and help to protect you

against the bad bacteria that put you at risk of gum disease and tooth decay.

When taken orally, the probiotics in the supplements are directly delivered to your mouth, allowing for easy colonization of your oral biofilms. There are some toothpastes on the market that contain probiotics. However, most dental probiotics come in the form of a chewable tablet, mouth rinse, lozenge or drink. While it would be ideal to get these through a mouthwash or rinse, studies have shown many of the probiotics will not integrate well with liquid on a long-term basis. The best way to get the proper oral probiotics would be with an effervescent tablet for mouthwash or a chewable tablet that you can rinse with Ozone water in order to kill the bad bacteria.

There are many different strains of bacteria. Here is a short list of a few and what they specialize with.

• One of the most problematic bacteria in the development of cavities is called Streptococcus mutans. However, an oral probiotic strain called Streptococcus A12 can outcompete the harmful version and prevent plaque buildup.

• At least 11 clinical trials show that oral probiotics may improve gum disease symptoms. The best oral probiotics for gum disease are:, L. reuteri, L. brevis.

- Oral thrush, or oral candidiasis, is a fungal condition in which candida fungus (usually C. albicans) overgrows and forms white spots on your tongue. Burning, redness, and dry mouth can occur. Oral/dental probiotics may prevent or help to reverse oral thrush. The best oral probiotics for oral thrush/candidiasis are: Lactobacillus spp. S. salivarius K12.

- Dental probiotics may stop bad breath by reducing the compounds which may cause halitosis. The best dental probiotics for bad breath include: S. salivarius K12, L. salivarius, L. reuteri, L. casei.

- Oral probiotics may reduce the risk of respiratory infections, particularly in children. The best oral probiotics for respiratory infections are: S. salivarius K12, S. salivarius M18, L. reuteri, L. sakei, L. paracasei, L. gasseri.

- Oral probiotics may reduce symptoms of recurrent tonsillitis. The best probiotic for tonsillitis is S. salivarius K12.

- According to two reviews published in 2020, oral probiotic strains capable of stopping oral cancer growth include: L. rhamnosus GG, L. plantarum, Acetobacter syzygii, and L. salivarius REN. More research is needed to draw serious conclusions, but there is no scientific evidence that oral probiotics can treat or reverse oral cancer in humans.

Many people wonder, should I take oral probiotics in the morning or at night? The best time to take oral probiotics is in the morning after finishing your oral hygiene routine. There is really no bad time to try and add more soldiers to fight for the health and wellbeing of your mouth, so do not hesitate to use the probiotics again throughout the day and get rid of some of those vicious bacteria.

Chapter 3:

Best toothpaste

This is where we get a little long winded, since we will be breaking down a few of the **poisons** -I mean ingredients- that are in 95% of today's toothpaste. I will go into a small history on a few things as it will be necessary to understand why we are still being slowly poisoned daily. Even with a somewhat detailed explanation, you will still wonder why this has not changed or even become a topic of consideration sooner. Toothpaste has a very long history, much longer than many people realize.

History

EGYPT

As far as we know, the first use of toothpaste can be dated back to 5000 BC by the Egyptians. The oldest toothpaste recipe was found in a collection of papyrus documents at the National Library in Vienna, Austria. According to the document, written in the fourth century AD, the ingredients needed for a happy white smile are, one drachma of rock salt - a measure equal to one-hundredth of an ounce - two drachmas of mint, one drachma of dried iris flower and 20 grains of pepper, all of them crushed and mixed.

It would have been a little rough on the gums, but a few dentists say that the formula is better than what we had to begin with. Further recipes were found consisting of powdered ashes from oxen hooves, myrrh, eggshells, pumice, and water (the actual "toothpaste" was likely a powder at first, with the water probably added at the time of use). After examining research of more than 3,000 mummies, anatomists and paleo pathologists at the University of Zurich concluded that 18 percent of all mummies in case reports showed a nightmare array of dental diseases. Worn teeth, periodontal diseases, abscesses and cavities tormented the ancient Egyptians, according to these

first studies performed on Egyptian
mummies. This would explain

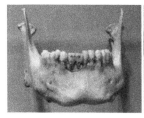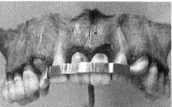

why they were determined to create a
paste that would eliminate this problem.
There were also toothpicks found next
to tombs, no doubt to remove food
debris the same way we try today.

ROME

The Roman leaders used iterations of
the Egyptian mixture but began
experimenting with their own
toothpaste. They added more abrasives

to their mixture so as to increase the cleaning power, the most popular of which were crushed bones and oyster shells. However, before doing this one of the more popular things the Romans used as mouthwash and to brush their teeth with was urine. They did have an intelligent basis behind this, it was not just because they wanted to taste their bodily fluids. Urine as we probably know contains ammonia, which in our present day and age we use as a cleaning agent. Another thing that Ammonia is capable of doing is whitening teeth and can help in preventing cavities. This was also something that everyone had and could use inexpensively. This also spurned many entrepreneurs such as laundrymen, to place a jar out in the front of their businesses so that anyone could just pee into it and help them turn a profit. Believed to be the strongest in the world and most effective, Portuguese urine was shipped in large quantities from Portugal for rich Roman ladies to use on their teeth. This was when emperors Nero and Vespasian both introduced urine taxes because they saw how much money these laundrymen were making and figured that they could easily make money off of people's bathroom breaks.

Some of the other controversial toothpaste recipes were from Pliny the Elder – He advised to prepare good "toothpaste" that included ashes, head of hare and donkey teeth, mixed with extracts of mouse brain or hair."

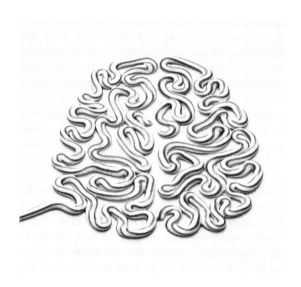

CHINA

It is said that a Chinese man named Huang Ti studied how to take care of teeth and then claimed that tooth aches could be cured by putting gold and silver needles in different parts of the jaw and gum.

The Chinese preferred natural ingredients in their toothpaste such as ginseng, mints, and salt. They developed chewing sticks — aromatic tree twigs — to get rid of buildup and freshen breath. No doubt this was a much better tasting toothpaste than that of the Egyptians, and I would say slightly better than the urine used by some of the Romans. One thing that was consistent in all areas for the most part was that if you had money, you had access to toothpaste, but if you were poor or had very little money you did not get quality toothpaste very often. In China they would also use bones and twigs and then mash them together with flower petals, salt, and water, to form a thick paste. They would then apply this paste on the end of a bamboo leaf to place it on the teeth.

Apart from toothbrushing, there were other ways that the Ancient Chinese would keep their teeth clean and breath smelling fresh. For instance, rinsing the mouth with tea after eating, using poria fungus as toothpaste, and sprinkling certain herbs or spices into one's mouth were also important for the Ancient Chinese.

After the recorded history of Chinese toothpaste and ingredients, there is a long gap before any types of advancement for toothpaste or oral hygiene products were documented. As these powders and pastes made it into the west, if you had money you would have access to these oral care products, but if you were poor you did not have access to them.

We see that in the early 1800's soap started to be added into these pastes. Starting in the 1850's was when we see the paste being sold in jars. Colgate finally came on the scene shortly after this with mass production in 1873. While these pastes scraped all the bad debris and bacteria from the teeth, it was also so abrasive that it would take off most of the enamel. This brings us to a point much closer to home, because in 1914 we finally started seeing our toothpaste sold in tubes, similar to how they are today. This is where things start getting interesting with the different ingredients being added. Toxic chemicals such as fluoride began to be introduced into our toothpaste.

TOXIC POISONS ADDED TO OUR TOOTHPASTE

Sodium Lauryl Sulfate

This is a synthetic, organic compound present in a great variety of industrial and personal care products. This chemical can serve as an emulsifier, foaming agent, detergent, and surfactant, or substance that reduces surface tension and allows better interaction between liquids and solids. These qualities, combined with the fact that sodium lauryl sulfate is quite cheap to make, has made it a popular ingredient in everything from shampoos to engine degreasers to laundry soaps.

Some concerns are that sodium lauryl sulfate can irritate the skin and eyes. Undiluted, this compound is an irritant, and even concentrations of just two percent can aggravate the eyes and skin. Rashes, dandruff, psoriasis, canker sores, cataracts, and dermatitis have all been linked to excess sodium lauryl sulfate exposure. Because of the above side effects, the International Journal of Toxicology has recommended sodium lauryl sulfate concentrations of no more than one percent.

The body is unable to break down this compound and excrete it like normal nutrients, but can instead absorb it. This means that sodium lauryl sulfate can accumulate within the body over a certain period, and that these residual levels can eventually become much higher. More than just causing skin inflammation, these trace amounts of sodium lauryl sulfate are able to disrupt the natural balance of hormones by mimicking hormones such as oestrogen, a type of estrogen.

Whether in its pure form or as part of a product, sodium lauryl sulfate is combustible and when heated it can emit irritating or toxic fumes.

These fumes can contain sulfur oxides, which are sharp-smelling gasses that can cause coughing, wheezing, and shortness of breath. Respiratory irritation may occur as well. Sodium lauryl sulfate should never be consumed. Ingesting this compound can result in an individual experiencing nausea, vomiting, and diarrhea.

Sodium lauryl sulfate, which is commonly found in personal care and beauty products, can be found in the following items:

TOOTHPASTE MOUTHWASH

Body Washes

Liquid Hand Soaps

Mascara

Moisturizers

Shampoos

Skin cleansers

Soaps

Sunscreen And Sunblock Lotions

Laundry Detergents

Stain Removers

Sodium lauryl sulfate is not something
to be taken in excess. With that being
said, I would not add anything to my

mouth that has been a toxic poison of any kind.

FLUORIDE

In the 1940's when the war was still going on, the main focus was how fast we could create nuclear weapons, which included the Atomic bomb. To create these weapons of mass destruction most people since then know that the main ingredient is Uranium. What they choose not to tell you, and for good reason, is that the second ingredient was Fluoride. Yes, the exact same Fluoride chemical that is added to most TOOTHPASTES, most WATER in the USA, as well as things such as ski wax, Teflon plastics, carpets, any types of WATERPROOF clothing, POPCORN bags, pesticides, HAMBURGER wrappers, and even PIZZA BOXES!!!! Fluoride was being manufactured at the time for the purpose of enriching the uranium in the nuclear weapons. The problem was how many factory workers were getting sick, as well as the local farmers and animals. Cows on the farm could not even stand to graze and eat. They had to crawl through the grass to eat, while the farmers stayed in their houses and puked violently from the fluoride particles in the air. All of this led to massive lawsuits which involved high name figures in the military that needed to make sure the manufacturing of Fluoride was never stopped or slowed down. This would be the first time the country would have to make a choice between "national security" and the actual wellbeing and safety of the American people. This choice decided the fate of every National security situation moving forward. Since then, most people have no idea that the Fluoride being added to our drinking water in the USA and many other things we use on a daily basis is actually an industrial waste that is scrubbed from the smokestacks of Florida phosphate fertilizer mills to prevent it from damaging livestock and crops in the surrounding countryside. This way, the phosphate companies do not need to pay for toxic waste removal. Instead, they just sell it to the municipalities and have it shipped all across North America to be added to our drinking water.

Here are a few things that have been studied and proven to be caused by Fluoride:

- A 12-year study determined lower I.Q in kids that had baby formula mixed with Fluoridated water.
- 400 studies that have determined Fluoride a neurotoxin.

- Fluoride turns your teeth yellow and brown.

- Cancer

- Diabetes

Heart disease

- Kidney disease

- Lower testosterone levels causing male infertility

- Thyroid disease

- Acute toxicity

- 65 human studies linking moderately high fluoride exposures to reduced intelligence.

These are all just little samples of some of the dangers we see with Fluoride consumption. The problem is that there is nobody to tell us how much is in our water or when we are drinking too much of it, especially in conjunction with all the other Fluoride added products. Our filtered water and bottled water have Fluoride, and it is very difficult to find filters that will actually filter out this poison. Fluoride is also known to make us much more docile and suggestible. With its ability to sterilize men and stop procreation, as well as weaken muscle and bone, if there is an altercation it would be almost impossible to eliminate the chances for serious injury. Amongst all the side effects mentioned prior, this is why it was the toxic substance of choice in WWII by Hitler. He knew that if given to the people they would not only be more likely to listen to everything they were told, but they would willingly accept it.

While it may be near impossible to eliminate this chemical completely from our everyday lives, there are a few ways we can start.

1. Start by using a PROPER water filter that can filter fluoride. They are not easy to find and can be a little pricey, but they do exist.

2. Eliminate this chemical COMPLETELY from all your oral products!!!!!

Instead of using toothpaste with fluoride, we should replace this with something all natural, vegan-friendly and healthy such as NANO SILVER. The history of NANO SILVER is extensive and can be traced back hundreds of years. It is used in multiple products and is even safe for babies. Brushing our teeth is the first thing we do to start our day and the last thing we do before we go to bed. Starting here would be the most ideal place. We really should be taking our oral care more seriously and thinking about it as more of an oral wellness by using products like NANO SILVER, or even healthy alcohol-free mouthwash. Maybe even adding Vitamin C and Elderberry as something that would boost your immune system early in the morning. These are not just ways in which we can eliminate poison from our lives, but active ways to replace it with something healthy that can help us function with more cognitive abilities while building our immune systems. So the next time your dentist tells you that fluoride is only bad if you have an overexposure to it, ask him or her, *How much Fluoride have YOU had today doc?*

Triclosan

Triclosan is an artificial antibacterial and antifungal agent (biocide) designed to help kill and reduce the growth of bacteria within the body and on the surface of the skin. It was created in 1964 by a Swiss pharmaceutical company (Ciba-Geigy). Since then, it has been included (in small amounts) in a variety of different domestic products such as soaps, shampoo, deodorants, toothpaste, mouthwashes, cleaning supplies and pesticides to name a few. It is also often included in consumer products such as kitchen utensils, toys, bedding, trash bags, and even socks.

If you are not yet aware of the potential dangers of triclosan, you should know that this antibacterial agent has been strongly linked to the following effects on human health:

* Abnormalities with the endocrine system, particularly with thyroid hormone signaling

* Weakening of the immune system

* Birth defects

* Uncontrolled cell growth

* Unhealthy weight loss

Therefore, the FDA has placed a ban on triclosan and all related antibacterial soap chemicals, with manufacturers having only one year to remove it and 18 other antibacterial ingredients from products.

Propylene Glycol

Propylene glycol is actually the mineral oils which are extensively used in the paints, enamels, antifreeze and airplane deicers in the industrial grade. While in its pharmaceutical grade, propylene glycol is found in many applications including personal care products such as toothpaste.

In toothpaste, this chemical is used as the surfactant. As mentioned before, surfactant is the chemical which has the role of forming the foam in the toothpaste. This harmful chemical has the risk of causing skin, lung, and eye irritation, and can possibly introduce toxins to the human organs. This is one of the harmful chemicals in toothpaste which you should avoid.

Propylene glycol enters the body as an alcohol and metabolizes in the body's enzyme pathways. These pathways do not mature in humans until 12 to 30 months of age. Infants and children below the age of 4 years, pregnant women, and those with kidney dysfunction or in renal failure are not able to eliminate propylene glycol in the body. Even the FDA concedes this inability to process and eliminate this product which causes potential adverse reactions in **infants** and **pregnant women** as well as those **with kidney problems**.

Diethanolamine or DEA

Diethanolamine is a chemical normally used because of its ability to foam. We all know that toothpaste tastes better and gives the illusion that it is working better if it is foaming up. Because of this thought process, many toothpastes use this chemical which is also known as the hormone disruptor. DEA can react with other ingredients or compounds that will create the carcinogenic compound called N-nitrosodiethanolamine or NDEA. This NDEA can infect your skin and possibly cause dreadful diseases like stomach, liver, bladder, and esophageal cancers. The Environmental Working Group has listed this chemical as a 10 in the cosmetic list. What this means is that DEA is considered one of the highest most toxic chemicals to the human body. It contains toxins which can attack human organs, cause irritation and cancer. This is a chemical that you want to make sure is not in your toothpaste.

This is a good start to some of the more dangerous chemicals that have been added since we have started our "toothpaste improvements" over the years. These days there are a few good all natural, vegan, and organic brands out there. Most have a hard time competing with the giants in the industry, even though they keep cancer causing, brain damaging, disease enhancing chemicals out of their products. A good rule of thumb is if it was used in the past for any types of poison, or has been proven by multiple parties to be damaging to your brain, organs or body, I choose to stay away. I believe there are a few very positive ingredients that can take over for some of these poisons.

TOOTHPASTE INGREDIENTS WE CAN USE INSTEAD OF POISON!

Baking Soda

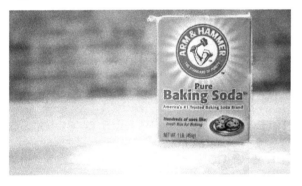

Baking soda, or sodium bicarbonate, is a fine, white powder with almost innumerable household uses. When you brush, grains of baking soda disrupt the biofilm, reducing the bacteria count and helping to prevent damage to your teeth and gums. Some harmful bacteria need more acidic conditions in order to thrive in your mouth. A 2017 study showed that when you rinse your mouth with a baking soda and water solution, the pH in your mouth increases, making it less acidic. As a result, using baking soda as a toothpaste may make it harder for cavity-causing bacteria to multiply in your mouth.

Baking soda has natural whitening properties and has been shown to be effective at removing stains on your teeth and whitening your smile. That's why it's a popular ingredient in many commercial toothpastes. Numerous studies have shown that baking soda is a mild abrasive that has the ability to remove stains from the outside of your teeth.

While the American Dental Association (ADA) considers baking soda safe for your enamel and dentin, some researchers have given it a low rating as a teeth whitener because it may not remove stains as effectively as some other products. If baking soda doesn't work well for you as a teeth whitener, you may want to consider products that contain hydrogen peroxide or microbead abrasives(not all natural).

For many users, the biggest downside of brushing with straight baking soda or a baking soda paste is that it doesn't taste very pleasant. Baking soda's texture may also make you feel like you have sand in your mouth. This is all based on using just baking soda and not paste.

NEEM

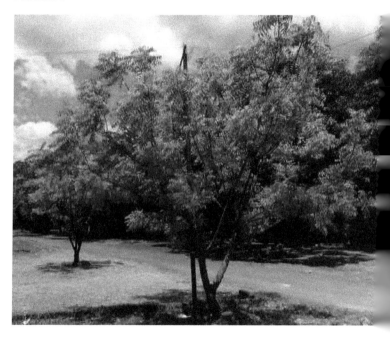

Neem oil is a traditional treatment for gums and teeth extracted from the evergreen neem plant found mostly on the Indian continent, where the twigs and leaves of the plant have been used to provide effective oral care for centuries. It is an anti-bacterial and anti-diabetic, a powerful antioxidant and astringent, and it possesses anti-inflammatory properties.

The ingestion of neem oil in large amounts has been shown to reduce fertility in limited animal studies. Women should avoid neem oil if they are pregnant or breastfeeding. These are some of the bad aspects of this age-old ingredient.

Charcoal

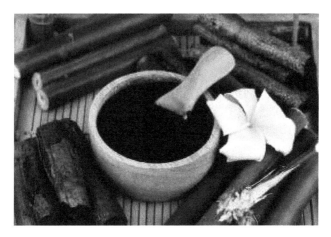

Activated charcoal — the type used in beauty products and toothpaste — is a fine grain powder made from wood, coconut shells, and other natural substances which are oxidized under extreme heat. It is highly absorbent and used medically to absorb and remove toxins. In order to whiten teeth, a product needs to work on stains on the surface, as well as intrinsic stains, which are those below the enamel.

Most charcoal toothpastes are too abrasive to be used on a regular basis, and using a material that's too abrasive on your teeth can wear down your enamel. This may make your teeth look more yellow by exposing the dentin, a calcified yellow tissue. It can also make your teeth more sensitive.

However, as long as you can find a charcoal that is less abrasive, it can be a good choice as a decent natural tooth whitening option. All the crazy potent adhesive qualities in those tiny pores help pull surface stains off your teeth (activated charcoal adsorbs tannins, a staining property found in coffee and wine) leaving you with a dazzling pearly white smile.

NANO SILVER

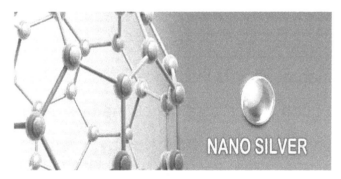

Silver has been used for at least six thousand years to prevent microbial infections. It has proven to be effective against almost all organisms tested, and has played an important role in the development of radiology and in improving wound healing, according to research out of the University of Cincinnati College of Medicine.

Before we were able to store our foods at cold temperatures, people would use silver coins in liquids to prevent bacterial growth. This is also the reason why we eat with "silverware" as we call it, even if the knife and fork are plastic. The term "silverware" comes from the fact that individuals would eat from actual silver so it would kill the bad bacteria before they placed the food in their mouths.

First, colloidal silver's ability to control antibiotic-resistant superbugs is second to none and unheard of. In the 1980's Dr. Ford documented over 650 different disease-causing pathogens that were destroyed in minutes when exposed to small amounts of silver. In case we are not aware, one of the biggest drawbacks with antibiotics is the fact that our bodies will adapt and become resistant to the antibiotics prescribed. The CDC has reported that an average of 23,000 people die from infections due to antibiotic resistance.

Colloidal silver however doesn't create resistance nor immunity in the organisms that are killed by it. What this is telling us is that the pathogens killed by silver will NOT adapt to it, and the silver continues to fight against the problem. With this being said, if silver is used as a toothpaste, the benefits can get into the bloodstream through the gums and help fight different types of bacteria as well as other pathogens besides tooth decay. Thanks to new technology, as of 2018, studies have shown GREAT benefits from being able to nanotize silver.

Colloidal silver is the perfect alternative to water in toothpaste. Since it is naturally antimicrobial and antibacterial, no preservatives are required to keep colloidal silver toothpaste fresh and safe. It also easily binds natural toothpaste ingredients together. Colloidal silver also works its way into the small pockets of your gum tissue called sulci. This is the tiny spot between where your teeth meet your gums. Bacteria can typically squeeze its way into the tiny sulci and trigger gum disease. Nano-silver gently cleanses a large majority of sulcus spaces to naturally remove dangerous bacteria and reduce inflammation. It has also been shown to eliminate tooth sensitivity since it is able to get into the pores of the teeth due to its size. It helps reduce and at times eliminate bleeding gums and bad breath (Halitosis). Silver has also been shown to boost the immune system, sometimes more effectively than Vitamin C.

Because of its rare ability to promote enamel growth, it can help to naturally whiten teeth.

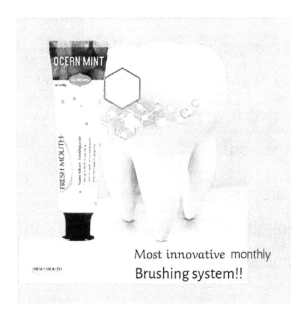

Most innovative monthly Brushing system!!

These are just a few of the amazing benefits of nano silver technology used in toothpaste as well as other areas of life. The benefits from Nano silver are enough to write an entire book on. However, the negatives are mostly companies upset and angry that fluoride is being eliminated, or people and companies unsure of how the Nano silver particles work. So, as you can see, there are many more healthy alternatives to the rat poisons which we have been brushing our teeth with.

There are also many different home-made toothpaste options you can try. Some are made with the above ingredients since they have so many antibacterial qualities.

1. ALL-NATURAL COCONUT OIL TOOTHPASTE

Ingredients:

2 tablespoons coconut oil (you can adjust the proportion based on your desired consistency)

1 tablespoon bentonite clay

1 teaspoon baking soda

1 teaspoon xylitol

2 teaspoons unsweetened cacao (optional) peppermint essential oil (optional)

Some of the benefits of **cacao powder** can be reduced inflammation, better blood flow, and lower blood pressure. Several studies have explored the protective effects of cocoa against dental cavities and gum disease.

Cocoa contains many compounds that have antibacterial, anti enzymatic and immune-stimulating properties that may contribute to its oral health effects.

In one study, rats infected with oral bacteria and were given cocoa extract had a significant reduction in dental cavities, compared to those given only water.

Coconut oil In particular, has been used in Ayurvedic medicine to clean and whiten teeth, reduce halitosis (bad breath), and improve gum health.

Directions:

In a small bowl, combine all the dry ingredients and mix it up! Pro-tip: it is best to use cocoa powder instead of bits you may need to crush.

Bit by bit, slowly add the coconut oil into the mixture. Keep mixing until you reach your desired texture and consistency.

Pour your homemade toothpaste into an empty container.

2. BAKING SODA TOOTHPASTE
Using baking soda regularly could help reduce the risk of gum

diseases like gingivitis, because it could prevent plaque formation and accumulation. When baking soda interacts with water or acid content, it will form bubbles that could help lift the stain, including the stains found in teeth.

Ingredients:

3 tablespoons coconut oil (certified organic)
3 tablespoons baking soda
½ teaspoon xylitol, stevia, or bentonite clay (optional)
5 drops essential oil like peppermint or tea tree (optional)

Directions:

Combine all the
ingredients in a small bowl
and mix. Keep mixing until
the mixture forms a paste.
To make things easier, you
may melt the coconut oil
first.
Use an airtight container to store
your homemade toothpaste.

3. Pink Himalayan salt toothpaste

The use of pink Himalayan salt in
toothpaste has been found to
offer superior plaque removal and
Gingivitis improvement. It also
helps fight bad breath and
eliminate teeth sensitivity.

Ingredients:

½ teaspoon Pink Himalayan mineral salt

4 tablespoons coconut oil

2-3 tablespoons of filtered water

4 tablespoons bentonite clay

10-15 drops peppermint essential oil

Directions:

In a small bowl, combine the coconut oil, clay, and salt.

Add one tablespoon of water to the bowl and use the back of a spoon to "cream" the mixture.

Keep adding in more water until it reaches your desired consistency.

Add the peppermint oil and keep mixing.

Pour your toothpaste into an airtight container.

4. Essential oils toothpaste

Essential oils may offer an all-natural and safe solution for the teeth whitening process, as well as pain relief. However, using essential oils for toothache pain must be done with caution. Never ingest essential oils, and always apply with caution. Read the instructions carefully and stop using essential oils for oral health if more pain or irritation is caused. Always consult your doctor before switching to anything that may be an irritation or may cause an allergic reaction.

Clove oil for tooth infection:
The potent antimicrobial and anti-inflammatory properties of clove essential oil have long been recommended as a powerful ingredient for all-natural mouthwash. According to one study, patients who used clove essential oil in their mouthwash had reduced plaque after four weeks of use. Because of its known antimicrobial and plaque-fighting qualities, it serves as one of the best essential oils for tooth infection.

Peppermint Oil for Toothache:
Using peppermint oil for teeth can be especially helpful for toothaches related to nerve pain. One notable benefit of peppermint essential oil is that it can soothe nerve pain and provide numbing relief when applied topically.

Eucalyptus Oil for Toothache:
When it comes to essential oils for an infected tooth or gums, eucalyptus essential oil should be at the top of the list. Two benefits of eucalyptus essential oil include its natural antibacterial and pain-relieving qualities.

Lavender Oils for Teeth Grinding

Lavender essential oil is one of the most popular scents in the world due to its wide variety of benefits.

It is perhaps best known for its calming effects when inhaled regularly. Reducing stress and inducing feelings of calmness may help reduce teeth grinding.

Lemon Essential Oil Teeth Whitening

It's also considered one of the most effective essential oils at preventing bacterial growth. The antibacterial properties will help maintain a healthy mouth.

The very nature of lemon also has some bleaching qualities,

which makes it among the best essential oils for teeth whitening.

Ingredients:

10 drops essential oil

5 tablespoons coconut oil

3 tablespoons baking soda

1 teaspoon sea salt or pink Himalayan salt

Directions:

In a small bowl, combine all the ingredients. To make things easier, you can soften up the coconut oil by warming it up first. Mix everything together.

Pour the mixture into an empty
container and seal it tightly.

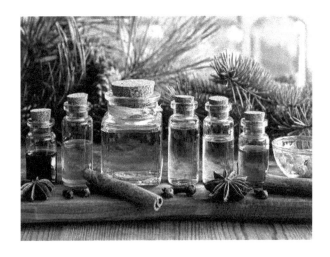

Chapter 4:

History of the

toothbrush

The first tooth cleaning instruments can be dated back to 3000B.C in ancient Babylonia, and were not exactly brushes but different types of chewed wood that people used to get food particles from between their teeth. There were different types of twigs used depending on geographic location, each of which typically had their own types of health and wellness benefits.

The bristle toothbrush, like the type used today, was not invented until 1498 in China when the king actually patented the invention. It was from this point that we followed the history of the toothbrush. The bristles were actually the stiff, coarse hairs taken from the back of a hog's neck or another similar animal and attached to handles made of bone or bamboo. It wasn't until 1938, that nylon bristles were used instead of animal hair by Dupont de Nemours.

Johnson & Johnson, a leading medical supplies firm, introduced the "Reach" toothbrush in 1977. It differed from previous toothbrushes in three ways:

1. It had an angled head, similar to dental instruments, for proper reach of the back teeth.

2. The bristles were concentrated more closely than usual to clean each tooth and rid the cavity causing bacteria more effectively.

3. The outer bristles were longer and
   softer than the inner bristles.

Other manufacturers soon followed with
other designs aimed at improving
effectiveness.

In the UK, William Addis is believed to
have produced the first mass-produced
toothbrush in 1780. In 1770, he was
jailed for causing a riot. While in prison,
he decided that using a rag with soot
and salt on the teeth was ineffective
and could be improved. After saving a
small bone from a meal, he drilled small
holes into the bone and tied into the
bone tufts of bristles that he had
obtained from one of the guards, then
passed the tufts of bristle through the

holes in the bone and sealed the holes with glue. After his release, he became wealthy after starting a business manufacturing toothbrushes. He died in 1808, leaving the business to his eldest son. It remained within family ownership until 1996. Under the name Wisdom Toothbrushes, the company now manufactures 70 million toothbrushes per year in the UK. By 1840, toothbrushes were being mass-produced in Britain, France, Germany, and Japan. Pig bristles were used for cheaper toothbrushes, while badger hair were for the more expensive ones.

In 1978 Dr. George C. Collis developed the Collis Curve toothbrush which was the first toothbrush to have curved bristles. The curved bristles follow the curvature of the teeth and safely reach in between the teeth and into the sulcular areas. Patented in 1985, curved bristles allow for safe and easy brushing of the teeth and gingival sulcus. In January 2003, the toothbrush was selected as the number one invention Americans could not live without according to the Lemelson-MIT Invention Index. This gives us a small insight into the few different ideas we have come up with for our toothbrushes.

1. Interdental brush

An interdental or proxy brush is a small brush, typically disposable, either supplied with a reusable angled plastic handle or an integral handle, used for cleaning between teeth and between the wires of dental braces and the teeth.

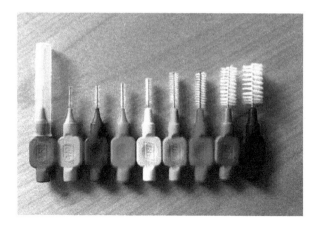

These brushes still come in a variety of heads, soft, medium, hard. Interdental brushes have a flexible neck for easier access, particularly to inaccessible areas between the back teeth. And do not worry if you bend the base of the wire during use, they will not break.

2. End-tuft brush

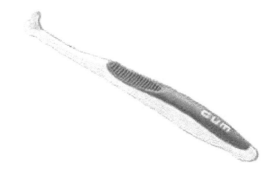

The small round brush head comprises seven tufts of tightly packed soft nylon bristles, trimmed so that the bristles in the center can reach deeper into small spaces.

It's very useful for smaller and harder to reach areas, and is also able to get into crevices behind the lower front teeth, the most common location for calculus build-up. The end-tuft brush reaches to the wisdom teeth more conveniently, removing food particles before a buildup causes infection. It also cleans around the margins of the crowns

3. Chewable toothbrush

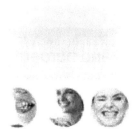

A chewable toothbrush is a miniature plastic molded toothbrush which can be placed inside the mouth. While not commonly used, they are useful to travelers and are sometimes available from bathroom vending machines. They are available in different flavors such as mint or bubblegum, and should be disposed of immediately after use. Other types of disposable toothbrushes include those that contain a small breakable plastic ball of toothpaste on the bristles, which can be used without water.

4. Electric toothbrush

SONIC VS ORAL-B

Electric toothbrushes can be classified, according to the speed of their movements such as: standard power toothbrushes, sonic toothbrushes, or ultrasonic toothbrushes. Any electric toothbrush is technically a power toothbrush. If the motion of the toothbrush is sufficiently rapid enough to produce a hum in the audible frequency range (20 Hz to 20,000 Hz), it can be classified as a sonic toothbrush. Any electric toothbrush with movement faster than this limit can be classified as an ultrasonic toothbrush. Certain ultrasonic toothbrushes, such as the Megasonex and the Ultreo, have both sonic and ultrasonic movements.

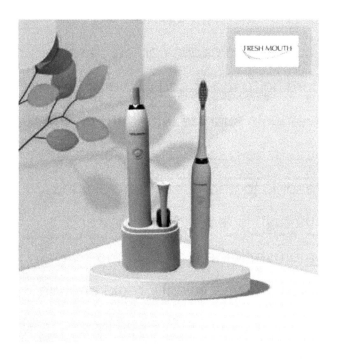

With all the different toothbrushes and options to reach your teeth in different angles, you must remember that you can also do damage depending on how you brush. It is beneficial, when using a straight bristled brush, not to scrub horizontally over the necks of teeth, not to press the brush too hard against the teeth, to choose toothpaste too abrasive, and to wait at least 30 minutes after consumption of acidic food or drinks before brushing. The best way to clean your teeth is to use as little pressure as possible, and to move your brush in small circular movements at a slight angle, half on the gum and half on the tooth. Cleaning the gum line is vital, as bacteria accumulates here and forms deposits.

SONIC:

The sonic brush comes with so many benefits such as *Benefits:*

- After three months of use, plaque was reduced by 21 percent and gingivitis by 11 percent in some studies.

- More helpful with those who have carpal tunnel, arthritis, and developmental disabilities.

- Built in times to make sure you are brushing each quadrant for the proper amount of time.

- Most have pressure sensors to make sure you are not pressing too hard while you are brushing.

- The sonic pulses do the large majority of the work, so you just slide the brush to the proper position.

When you are purchasing a sonic brush, you want to keep a few things in mind. The most important thing is that it is NOT powered by disposable batteries!!! In most cases disposable batteries will NOT be strong enough to get the brush to a true sonic level. This means you have a really expensive "vibrating toothbrush" and NOT a sonic toothbrush. Many people think they have a good sonic brush because it vibrates, but don't realize that they just paid $20 to $40 dollars for a manual brush that should have been $3. Some say that it's okay because they wanted it for the timer to make sure they are brushing long enough. I myself would just buy a timer for a few dollars and not worry about the timer being attached to the brush.

ORAL-B

ORAL-B and sonic brushes do share many of the same benefits such as

- More helpful with those who have carpal tunnel, arthritis, and developmental disabilities.
- Built in times to make sure you are brushing each quadrant for the proper amount of time.

- Most have pressure sensors to make sure you are not pressing too hard while you are brushing.
- Some now have water that comes out while you brush

While there are a few similarities, and both brushes do give you a great clean feeling, there is one thing you might want to pay attention to before deciding on which you should purchase.

Studies have shown that the ORAL-B can be more abrasive on the enamel depending on the person and how hard they brush. When the head does move on its own and the person brushing still brushes as hard or harder than normal, it can scrape at the enamel.

Fortunately, both sonic and oral-B have added pressure sensors to their newer brushes to help eliminate this problem. So no matter which one you decide to get, just remember that they both give better results and you should always pay attention to the pressure sensors and not brush too hard.

5. Bamboo toothbrush

Bamboo toothbrushes have soft nylon bristles that are comfortable and gentle against the teeth, but at the same time are firm for effective removal of plaques and stains from tea, coffee, red wine and food dye. The most widely known and popular advantage, a bamboo-based toothbrush, eliminates unnecessary waste while giving you the same quality of cleaning that a plastic brush can offer. Both the packaging and tossing of your toothbrush -recycling, reusing, or composting has never been easier. Another advantage of bamboo is that it is naturally antimicrobial. There's a reason cutting boards and kitchen utensils are made from wood and bamboo. Unlike plastic, properties inside the bamboo kill bacteria that penetrate its surface, providing long-lasting protection against harmful bacteria.

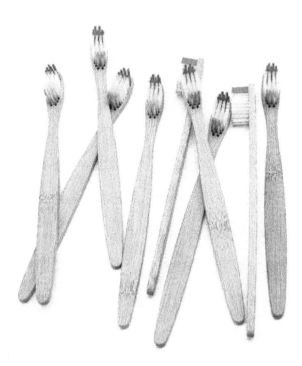

HOW OFTEN SHOULD WE CHANGE OUR BRUSH?

There have been many studies done on how long we should use our toothbrush before replacing it. There are a few factors that we want to bear in mind. Toothbrushes were found to be extensively contaminated with a variety of microorganisms after just a few weeks of use. Some of these are

- Pseudomonas which can cause suppurative otitis, eye infection, urinary tract infection, and burn infection.
- S. mutans cause initiation of dental caries

- lactobacilli cause *progression* of dental caries
- E-coli which in case you didn't realize is poop

This is just a few of the very many microorganisms that can be found after just a few weeks. After a few weeks, the bristles can also start to fray which will cause micro-tears in our gums and allow all those bad bacteria into our bloodstream wreaking havoc on our immune system. So it is not just our teeth that can be affected by poor oral hygiene, but an old brush can also make us surprisingly sick.

The types of bristles are of great importance as well. There are many people who feel that if they use a stronger, harder brush, that they will get more plaque off their teeth, or it will make their teeth whiter. The truth is, if your bristles are too hard, it can cause your gums to bleed, allowing that bad bacterium (E-coli/poop) into your bloodstream. One of the biggest problems using medium or hard bristle brushes is that it causes receding gums. If your gums begin to recede, you will notice that your teeth will begin to feel longer, there may be bleeding after brushing or flossing, bad breath, or loose teeth resulting in your teeth possibly falling out if you don't get it treated at your dentist. Basically, if you're using medium or hard bristle brushes your teeth could fall out after being humiliated with bad breath and bleeding gums. Yes, it is true that soft bristles will wear down faster, but this is not a problem if you are replacing the brush every month as suggested. Whether you use an electric brush or manual, this is true either way. You should replace your toothbrush every single month. Your health can be affected by this choice.

Here is a step by step on the proper ways of brushing your teeth given by a few different holistic dentists.

- *Angle the brush at 45 degrees*
  When brushing the sides of your teeth, tilt your brush 45 degrees

so that the bristles can reach inside the small gap between your teeth and gums. If plaque builds up in this pocket, it can lead to gum disease.

- *Brush gently with small circular motions*

small circular movements are the most effective and less damaging as opposed to brushing your teeth back-and- forth in a scrubbing motion. You also don't need to exert a lot of pressure, or scrub as hard as you can. Gentle pressure is enough to loosen plaque as stated earlier, because of the horrible problems it is capable of causing.

- *Brush every surface of every tooth*
  The order in which you brush your teeth doesn't matter, but doing it the same way every time can help ensure you don't miss any surfaces. This is one example of how you can brush your teeth:
- Begin at the back of your mouth, top left or top right
- Work your way around the outer surface of each tooth, brushing each one in small circular motions for a few seconds

- Turn your brush to the inner surface and work your way around the top again

- Brush the biting surface of your top molars and the back surface of your rear teeth

- Turn the brush vertically and use a downwards motion to brush the back of your front teeth a few times

- Repeat for the bottom teeth

- After cleaning your teeth, brush or scrape your tongue a few times

Another way is to break your mouth into four quadrants and spend 30 seconds on each one, brushing the inner, outer, and biting surfaces as you go. We only get one set of teeth, so always remember one thing while you are brushing your teeth....*"ONLY BRUSH THE ONES YOU WANT TO KEEP"*

CHAPTER 5

MOUTHWASH

Mouthwash dates back to ancient China, Egypt, Greece and Rome. Over the centuries, people tried different ingredients and combinations to get a healthy, good smelling mouth. These combinations included tortoise blood, milk, wine, olives, myrrh, fruits, and vinegar. Some have recommended a vigorous rinse with cold water to get rid of plaque and tartar. In the 1860's Dr. Joseph Lister began to develop the mouthwash people still use today.

Mouthwash can be used for many different reasons such as to treat infections, reduce inflammation, relieve pain, and reduce halitosis (bad breath). The preventive use of mouthwash is mainly to control the formation of cavities, and the therapeutic use is to help reduce bad bacteria that will destroy the oral microbiome, leading to plaque and other oral problems. Good oral health usually involves 3 steps: brushing, flossing, and rinsing. I am quite certain there are many people who do not rinse with mouthwash. Based on some of the different ingredients, this might be a good step to try and avoid. However, if you are using the proper mouthwash, it can be something that will change your life forever.

We will look in a little more detail about the history of mouthwash. There have been so many different, strange things people have done to keep their mouths clean, even besides swishing their mouths with urine. In the year A.D 23 the Romans would use tortoise blood as mouthwash because they thought it would disinfect their mouths and clean teeth. As time went by, they apparently wanted to do away with the blood idea and decided to do simpler things such as drinking goat's milk or rinsing with white wine.

In 70 A.D About two thousand years ago, Pedanius Dioscorides, a physician traveling throughout the Roman Empire, would collect samples of the local medicinal herbs everywhere he went. He turned his passion for plants and other medicinal substances into what we would call the encyclopedia on herbs and pharmacy that remained the supreme authority on the subject for 1,500 years. This is where he came up with a mixture of olive leaves, pickled olive juice, milk, pomegranate peelings, vinegar, and nutgalls as an effective treatment to reduce bad breath.

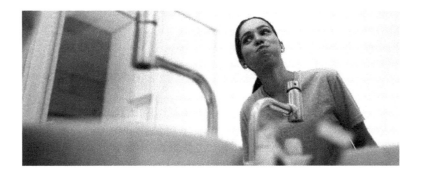

In the 12th century Saint Hildegard von Bingen, suggested that swishing pure, cold water around in the mouth can help remove tartar and plaque. This was a basic idea which lasted until the 16th century were Medieval oral hygiene practices centered around a mint and vinegar rinsing solution

were believed to rid the mouth of bad breath and germs.

In the 17th century Anton van Leeuwenhoek, a microscopist, discovered deposits on the teeth, which we now know as dental plaque which consists of living organisms. After some experimenting, van Leeuwenhoek discovered that using a mixture of vinegar and brandy would immediately kill organisms found in water, but for some reason would not kill those found in the mouth. His theory was that the mixture either did not reach the bacteria, or did not stay in the mouth long enough to affect the bacteria.

This meant trying to find a substance that could stay long enough in the mouth to attach and kill the bacteria. Harald Loe in the 1960's who was a professor in Denmark, used a chlorhexidine compound to prevent the buildup of plaque in the mouth. Chlorhexidine is effective because it adheres strongly to oral surfaces, and therefore, can remain present in the mouth for long durations while still being effective. This is how mouthwash as we know it was born.

This brings us to the mouthwash we are using currently. Most of us like to assume that when we change a formula of a product we are naturally enhancing its effectiveness and it must be better than the old outdated formula. I am here to tell you, and I believe others would agree, that this is **NOT** always the case. Some of the ingredients in our mouthwash today are dangerous to say the least. Let's just touch on two of the most common dangerous ingredients, one of which is misleading the world to think it is the best possible thing for our mouths.

Methyl salicylate:

is an organic compound with the formula C6H4(OH)(CO2CH3). It is the methyl ester of salicylic acid. It is a colorless, viscous liquid with a sweet, fruity odor reminiscent of root beer, but often associatively called "minty," as it is an ingredient in mint candies. It is produced by many species of plants, particularly wintergreens. It is also produced synthetically, used as a fragrance and a flavoring agent.

POSSIBLE SIDE EFFECTS:

BLADDER AND KIDNEYS:

Kidney failure --
decreased or no
urine output **EYES,**

EARS, NOSE, AND THROAT:

Eye irritation -- burning, redness, tearing, pain, light sensitivity

Loss of vision (from ulcers of the cornea)

Ringing in the ears

Throat swelling

LUNGS AND AIRWAYS:

Difficulty breathing

No breathing

Rapid breathing

NERVOUS SYSTEM:

Agitation, confusion, hallucinations

Coma (decreased level of consciousness and lack of responsiveness)

Deafness

Dizziness

Drowsiness

Headache

Fever

Seizures

STOMACH AND INTESTINES:

Nausea

Vomiting, possibly bloody.

Yes, you would need to swallow the mouthwash for some of these side effects to occur. However, some of these things can take place with the Methyl salicylate being absorbed through the gums, especially if you have an older, frayed toothbrush that when used creates micro-tears in the gums allowing more to transfer into the bloodstream through the gums. The next ingredient is the one we all think is most needed for mouthwash to be effective.

THE DANGERS OF ALCOHOL IN MOUTHWASH

Most people experience a burning sensation when they rinse their mouths with mouthwash, only to feel a sense of excitement and eagerness to finally spit it out, all for that fresh minty, clean feel in their mouths. Most people think "no pain, no gain" believing that the more it burns, the more effective the mouthwash is. Unfortunately, it appears that not only is alcohol not necessary for a mouthwash to be effective, but it may also even be detrimental to your oral health. Most of us have always believed that alcohol is added to mouthwash for the purpose of killing bacteria, and while the alcohol does kill ALL bacteria both BAD and GOOD, this is supposedly not the real reason based on certain studies. The alcohol is meant to act as a carrier agent for the active ingredients like eucalyptol, menthol, and thymol. It is these active ingredients that are responsible for penetrating plaque. This is a fact that Crest has put on their own website.

Many leading brands of mouthwash contain alcohol, and finding out the exact content of alcohol in your mouthwash can help you understand the risks if you drink it. Finding out the exact alcohol content in different brands of mouthwash can help you avoid an unintended conviction for drunk driving and help reduce the risks that are thought to be associated with mouthwashes having high alcohol content. Here are a few interesting facts to consider. Beer has between 3 and 8 percent alcohol, wine has around 12 percent, and spirits such as rum, whisky and vodka have around 40 percent.

Listerine Antiseptic

Listerine is one of the most well-known brands of mouthwash, and also has one of the highest percentages of alcohol. The alcohol content of ordinary Listerine is 26.9 percent: this is more than three times the content of beer. Some different varieties of Listerine have an alcohol content of as low as 21 percent. Listerine hit the news in 2005 when a driver was arrested for driving under the influence after quaffing three glasses of Listerine before heading out in the car. She ran into the back of another car at a stop light and failed a breathalyzer test when it was issued.

• Listerine is one of the most well-known brands of mouthwash and has one of the highest percentages of alcohol.

- Listerine hit the news in 2005 when a driver was arrested for driving under the influence after quaffing three glasses or Listerine before heading out in the car.

Colgate Mouthwash

Colgate mouthwash has a lower alcohol content than Listerine, but still contains 15.3 percent alcohol, almost double the amount of the strongest beer. This is more than most bottles of wine, so despite the much lower percentage, caution should still be exercised when making use of this mouthwash. Some researchers believe that mouthwash which contains alcohol increases the risk of developing oral cancers (as alcohol does); particularly because mouthwash is swilled around in the mouth, giving the alcohol a longer period of time to be absorbed into the cheeks.

Cepacol/Cepacol Mint

Cepacol brand mouthwashes contain a slightly lower amount of alcohol than Colgate, coming in at 14.5 percent. This is still stronger than many bottles of wine, so spitting the mouthwash out is advised. Many people believe children are particularly at risk from the alcohol content in mouthwash, with some risk of death for younger children. According to Dr. Dan Peterson of Family Gentle Dental Care, children weighing 26 pounds or less can be at risk of death after consuming 5 to 10 oz. of alcohol-containing mouthwash.

- Cepacol brand mouthwashes contain a slightly lower amount of alcohol than Colgate, coming in at 14.5 percent.

- Many people believe children are particularly at risk from the alcohol content in mouthwash, with some risk of death for younger children.

Another study conducted by Werner and Seymour analyzed data from multiple studies comparing alcohol to non-alcohol mouthwash concluded that "the alcohol component of mouthwashes affords little additional benefit, especially since it also kills the good bacteria that is there to protect you, or to enhance the other active ingredients in terms of plaque and gingivitis control".

ALCOHOL MOUTHWASH EFFECTS:

- **Halitosis (which is dry mouth)** After using mouthwash with alcohol, your mouth produces much less saliva. With no saliva to wash the bad bacteria off your teeth, your mouth now encourages **BAD** bacterial growth. By doing this on a regular basis it will ironically worsen your breath. So, if it is a fresh breath you are trying to accomplish with mouthwash, the alcohol will actually give the opposite reaction and your breath will continue to worsen.

· **CANCER**

This is not proven completely, as the premise and current studies behind it are assumed to be because of smokers. Many smokers and heavy drinkers often use mouthwash to try and mask their breath. After using the alcohol in the mouthwash, the cigarette smoke can more easily get into the bloodstream.

- **ALCOHOLISM**

  When someone has had a battle with alcoholism and is now trying to stay sober, it is best to stay away from these alcohol based mouthwashes despite what the companies and their paid-off scientists tell you. The fact of the matter is that there is almost 3 times more alcohol in the mouthwash than there is in some of the strongest beers, so common sense should say that this is probably **NOT** the best idea to try. These are just a few different things we need to be concerned about when using alcohol-based mouthwash. So, in the last few decades some can make the argument that we have made mouthwash worse than in the years past. Well, it might not be quite as bad as swishing around other people's urine in your mouth, but it definitely has not improved upon in the last few years. However as of late there have been many healthier alternatives available which are alcohol-free.

Therapeutic Mouthwash

Most people are trying to use mouthwash while out at dinner or on a date to quickly cover up bad breath from the last meal or drink they had, not really caring what kind of bacteria it is killing or what damage may be occurring. The only objective is to eliminate the bad breath now and worry about any type of consequences later. Therapeutic mouthwash is much different, as it is not only trying to eliminate the bad breath, but it kills the bacteria, which leads to bad breath while reducing plaque, gingivitis (gum disease), and cavities. It is much more of a wellness product, fighting against and/or helping to cure the things which caused the problem in the first place. The regular use of mouthwash stops cavities from forming around your gums. This will also prevent the build-up of bacteria in hard-to-reach places.

Therapeutic Mouthwashes contain active ingredients such as Nanosilver, probiotics and others that help to eliminate bacteria which in turn reduces gingivitis, cavities, plaque, and bad-breath. Be careful while buying some of these products as they may still try using harmful neurotoxins such as Fluoride. Remember, this was used for the atomic bomb and rat poison. There are many other problems with fluoride, but I think you will remember those two things as good reasons to stay away from it. Some of the best things to look for with therapeutic mouthwash is oil pulling, because most people that support oil pulling will only do so if it is done in an all-natural way.

OIL PULLING

Puneet Nanda, the creator of GuruNanda Pulling Oil, said oil pulling is supposed to get rid of oil-soluble toxins and harmful bacteria that build up in the mouth. This is done by swishing different types of oil in your mouth for 5 to 30 minutes, depending on the situation and the types of oil being used. Sunflower oil and sesame oil were some of the first ones that the original practitioner used close to 3000 years ago in India. Oil pulling was thought to not only prevent dryness of the throat, bleeding gums, and cracked lips, but it could also strengthen the teeth, gums, and jaw. It is described as a natural healing method for oral health, using chewing sticks and eating herbs in addition to the oils. Different oils can have different physical benefits besides just healing and protecting our gums.

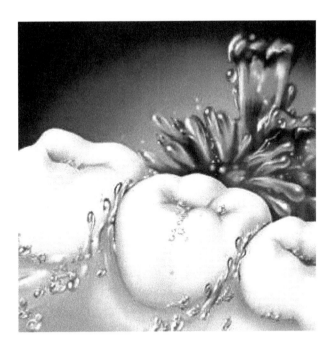

How to do the oil pulling activity?

- The stomach must be empty for at least 2 hours prior to doing oil pulling activity. So, the morning period is ideally better for doing it.

- After putting the oil in the mouth, it must be gargled for around 10 minutes. Make sure all the areas of the mouth are covered properly while doing this activity.
- Once you do it, spit it out totally. Make sure
- you do not swallow the oil after gargling it as it contains different bacteria and toxins from the mouth.
- Do this activity around 3 to 4 times with each activity being done for around 10 minutes.
- After the completion of the oil pulling activity, the mouth must be rinsed properly with the solution of warm and saltwater. It will

remove all the bacteria and other toxins from the mouth.

- Finally, after doing oil pulling, you can do the brushing activity properly.

DIFFERENT OILS

SESAME OIL: The antioxidant property and lots of Vitamin E present in the sesame oil are helpful for the removal of the bacteria. This oil has the capacity to loosen the plaque to further aid complete plaque removal.

COCONUT OIL: Coconut oil is one of the most popular oils used for oil pulling. Some choose to warm this oil slightly before putting it in the mouth. Gargling it properly can be instrumental in cleaning all the bacteria and other germs from the mouth. It is also one of the safest choices as it has no harmful effects if swallowed and digested.

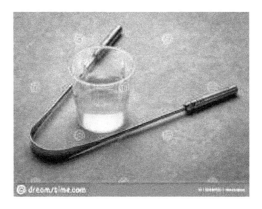

SUNFLOWER OIL: Sunflower oil is an acquired taste, so there are many people that choose not to use this as their first choice. The gargling can be done for 5 minutes properly which helps to loosen up the plaque and remove it from the teeth.

OLIVE OIL: Olive Oil has some antibacterial and antiviral properties that make it more suitable for oil pulling activity. These oils have shown some nice results in the removal of the plaque and tartar from the teeth.

Should I rinse with Hydrogen Peroxide?

Lately one of the most popular questions that I have heard is, should I rinse with hydrogen peroxide? Or that someone is already rinsing with Hydrogen

Peroxide. As with most of the things in the health and wellness industry that deal with our body, there are great benefits as well as great side effects if you do not know what products to use, why, or how to use these products. Hydrogen Peroxide is one of the main ingredients in home teeth whitening kits. Is this a healthy choice for a daily mouthwash that I would feel comfortable recommending to someone I care about? Let's look at the good and the bad.

Benefits:

Some of the benefits that do come with Hydrogen Peroxide according

to a few different scientific reports
are.....

1. **SOOTHING SORE THROATS**

Has antibacterial properties which
help your body fight off infections
that cause sore throats. It also helps
hardened or thick mucus in your
throat loosen and drain better,
relieving irritation.

2. **TREATING GUM DISEASE**

A study in Scientific Reports found
that HP made participants' gums
healthier and reduced amounts of
the periodontal pathogen
Porphyromonas gingivalis, which
causes gingivitis.

3. HEALING CANKER SORES

Hydrogen Peroxide is antiseptic, and an antiseptic can help heal cuts and canker sores. When applied to a cut or sore, the Hydrogen Peroxide foams and releases oxygen, which helps clean the area and reduce bacteria.

Most would say that these are great reasons to use Hydrogen Peroxide as your new mouthwash of choice. With these benefits as well as the added fact of it whitening your teeth, I would normally agree that it might be time to consider making the switch. However, before making the big jump into this supposedly miraculous rinse let's look at the downside, and I believe afterwards most of you will agree it is not the best choice.

Negative effects:

1. HARMFUL WHEN INGESTED

Swallowing too much Hydrogen Peroxide can cause serious side effects, including burning of the digestive tract, nausea, and vomiting.

2. BLACK HAIRY TONGUE

Yes healthwise this is not a serious condition, and it looks much worse than it really is since it is only temporary. However, the thought of this being my tongue is enough to make me never ever allow Hydrogen Peroxide near my mouth.

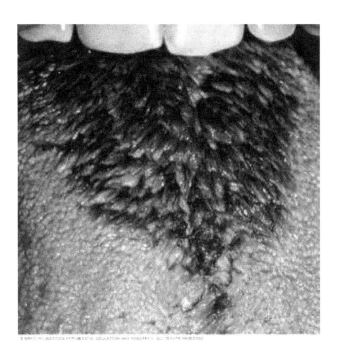

3. WEAKENED ENAMEL

While the black hairy tongue is enough for me to give up on the idea of using Hydrogen Peroxide, this is probably the best reason. Hydrogen peroxide can damage tooth enamel if used for too long, too often, or in too high concentrations. The reason for this is because it can penetrate the enamel, dentin, and collagen-rich tissue found within the dentin, damaging it as a result. This would not be my first choice for a mouth rinse.

There are also different recipes that will give you a healthier mouthwash option. If you decide to try any of these you should contact your doctor to make sure you do not have any types of allergic reactions to any of the ingredients. Here is a list of a few different options.

1. **Sage and salt mouthwash**
Sage is on the top of the list of recipes to improve oral and dental health, because of its anti-inflammatory and antibacterial properties. Many oral and dental diseases have been treated by various Sage preparations.

Ingredients:
Filtered Water
1 tsp of mineral Rich Salt
Organic sage leaves

Method –

In a bottle, put 6 sage leaves inside.

Dissolve salt in 5 oz. of boiling water.

After all is dissolved, pour boiling water inside the bottle.

use daily after brushing your teeth, until mouthwash is finished or continue a little longer if your oral health still is not up to scratch.

2. Salt and baking soda

This mouthwash is great for those who want to treat and

cure the cold and flu as well as other viral infections.

Ingredients:

1/2 spoon of Baking soda

1/2 spoon of salt

1 Cup of water

Method –

Mix baking soda and salt with water and use after brushing the teeth. Rinse your mouth well for 2 to 5 minutes and you will notice your teeth have a much stronger shine.

3. Herbal mouthwash

natural herbal mouth rinse is healthy for your mouth, teeth, and gums....and even contains nutrients for general health.

Ingredients:

4 oz of peppermint and sage leaves plus Echinacea Angustifolia root

8-12 drops of mint extract

1   tsp of thyme

2   tsp of Myrrh gum extract

5-7 drops of eucalyptus oil

Method –

Prepare a herbal infusion with the peppermint leaves, sage leaves and Echinacea Angustifolia, and then take a mason jar and pour all the ingredients together in it. Keep shaking strongly until blended well, and you are done.

4. Lemon juice and water

Lemon is highly antibacterial, as it improves vitamin C levels, can Alkalize Our pH, and can boost metabolism. Its antibacterial properties make it a great choice for fighting against plaque.

Ingredients

1 glass of Warm water

1 lemon

Method –

Take the lemon and squeeze it into 1 glass of warm water and rinse your mouth and then spit it out.

5. Apple cider vinegar mouthwash

Apple cider vinegar has been reported to be a natural teeth whitener and bad breath neutralizer. So, it will certainly improve your oral and dental health.

Ingredients

2 tsp apple cider vinegar

1   cup of salt

1-2 drops of Vanilla essential oil

Method –

Mix and store in a jar. Swish your mouth with this solution!

It is important to note that a lot of homemade mouthwash recipes to improve oral and dental health may include salt, baking soda and or essential oils. This is because salt is a natural antibacterial, baking soda has been reported to whiten teeth naturally, and essential oils have antibacterial and anti - inflammatory properties, making them a powerful ingredient that can not only help improve oral and dental health, but also treat fungal infections and even boost immunity. Some of these ingredients may not work for everyone, and you may need to consult your doctor before trying any of these homemade solutions.

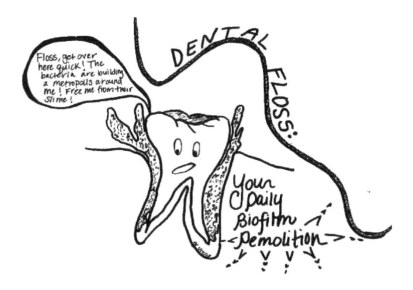

Chapter 6:

Benefits of dental floss

Dental floss is a thin string that has been in use for many years to remove food and dental plaque from between teeth in areas that a toothbrush is unable to reach. Most dentists recommend flossing as a preventative measure to avoid gingivitis and buildup of plaque. While there has been no real strong evidence, the ADA claims that flossing eliminates 80% of plaque.

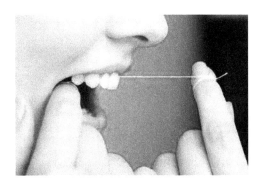

HISTORY

It is believed in archeological circles that there were markings on the teeth of found skulls that people used to floss in prehistoric times. However, in more modern times, in New Orleans, Levi Spear Parmly invented the first form of dental floss in 1815 and recommended that people clean their teeth with it daily. It wasn't until 1882 Codman and Shurtleft began manufacturing the first commercial dental floss from unwaxed silk that was available to the public in more mass amounts. In 1898 Johnson & Johnson took the same silk material used by doctors for silk stitches and were able to get the first patent on dental floss, even though Red Cross, Salter Sill Co. and Brunswick made their own brands of dental floss at the same time.

Despite these different companies trying to race to make their own brands of floss, and it being made ready to the common consumer across the country, it still did not catch a strong following until the 1940s. Because of the exorbitant costs of World War II Dr. Charles C. Bass invented nylon floss, and he found that it had greater abrasion resistance and elasticity than silk while at the same time being more readily available. With nylon floss, they were also able to add a wax coating over it, so that it was more comfortable to use without damaging the gums. Truth be told, many doctors have said that if you choose not to floss you choose not to clean 40% of your teeth. Even if you are a strong brusher, you will still miss 40% with brushing alone. Plaque and tartar buildup along your gum line is the fun result when you neglect cleaning that large portion of your teeth. Once you have this plaque it is usually not easy to remove, and this is an extensive task that is typically undertaken only by your dental hygienist. Infections in the gums can become prevalent when you do not floss on a regular basis, making the gums much more prone to bleeding. A lot of people like to claim that they do not floss because it makes their gums bleed, when in reality their gums bleed because they don't floss. Food particles and bacteria stay between your teeth and grow into damaging infections; add this to your bleeding gums and if you are not getting rid of your filthy toothbrush after one month you can be allowing toxic chemicals into your bloodstream. You should be flossing every day to remove potential causes of infection from your teeth.

Is your floss toxic?

Sadly, just like our toothpaste, there are many different dental flosses that have toxic chemicals added to them. As we have spoken about it earlier, one of the most toxic chemicals is fluoride. This neurotoxin has been the cause of many cancers, brain problems, among a long list of others. There is a chemical called Polytetrafluoroethylene (PTFE) which is derived from fluoride. We call this TEFLON, and we use it to make our non-stick pans, and waterproof clothing. It is extremely toxic, and this is a main ingredient in many different dental flosses. The dangers of this entering our bloodstream are much higher as our gums can bleed while flossing, allowing this heavily toxic substance into our system.

Teflon exposure has been linked to:

Hormone imbalance:

Hormones are chemicals produced in your endocrine glands. These powerful chemicals travel around your bloodstream instructing your tissues and organs on what to do. They basically organize, coordinate, and delegate the control of your body's major processes, including metabolism and reproduction.

Cancer

Cancer comes from overproduction, malfunction, and uncontrolled growth of abnormal cells anywhere in the body.

Autoimmune disease

On a normal basis a healthy immune system would defend the body against disease and infection. However, if the immune system malfunctions or is compromised in any way, it can mistakenly attack healthy cells, tissues, and organs. These attacks can affect any part of the body, weakening bodily function and even turning life-threatening. Scientists know of at least 80 types of autoimmune diseases. Some of these are type 1 diabetes, multiple sclerosis, lupus, and rheumatoid arthritis.

Neurotoxicity and Alzheimer's disease

Alzheimer's disease is basically senile dementia. A prominent cause of dementia is neurotoxicity. Neurotoxicity occurs when the exposure to natural or manmade toxic substances (neurotoxicants) alters the normal activity of the nervous system.

Some of the other types of materials used to make up our normal day-to-day dental floss are made from petroleum-based products. Health effects from exposure to petroleum products vary depending on the concentration of the substance. Breathing petroleum vapors can cause nervous system effects (such as headache, nausea, and dizziness) and respiratory irritation. Extremely high exposure can cause coma and death. Some of these basic materials are.....

1. Nylon

2. Polyester

3. Certain wax

This may all sound much more dangerous than it might be, considering the amounts being used in your dental floss. Let's just bear in mind that whatever goes into your mouth will go into your body, possibly your bloodstream with a chance of passing through your blood brain barrier which will affect you in all sorts of horrific ways, especially if our immune system is low. So, if there are any areas in our lives that we can mitigate the use of some of these substances, do you not agree that we should try to take advantage of this safe and healthy opportunity?

Some healthy alternatives are using a natural silk floss or a floss that is coated in a beeswax instead of petroleum-based wax. Another option is to use a water pik. This is considered by most to be one of the best, most effective ways of flossing. With this being said, you might want to consider the cost of the water pik. This can be the most expensive way to floss when you consider the cost of the unit.

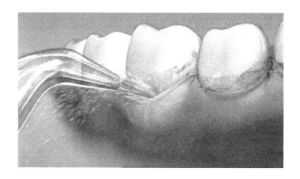

Is Water Flossing as Good as Dental Floss?

The American Dental Association says water flossers with the ADA Seal of Acceptance can get rid of plaque. It is quite interesting that they have made this statement because it may come across to some that the ADA might be trying to sell the specific units they choose to slap their seal of approval on, especially when they have no proven testing on some of the "chosen ones". Digging a little deeper into this, you may also notice that some studies find that water flossers *don't* remove plaque as well as traditional floss.

Water flossing has its place when it comes to certain circumstances in a person's life. A water flosser may be something you want to consider if you have trouble using dental floss. If you have braces or dental work like permanent or fixed bridges, a water flosser might be helpful. They can be good for people with periodontal disease or with extremely dry mouths. You might also want to try one if you have arthritis or other problems using your hands. Kids or teens with braces sometimes find water flossing easier than traditional flossing.

As long as we are trying to stay safe and are using the proper floss that is not laced with poison, there are definitely some very important benefits. The ADA states that some of the benefits of flossing on a daily basis are.

1. Removing plaque

If you are reaching areas that are not being reached with your brush you are preventing the build-up of plaque, which is a sticky coating which forms on your teeth. Plaque is colorless, so it is easy to allow this to grow without noticing. If you leave plaque, it will harden and turn into tartar, which is a yellow or brown color. Once you have tartar on your teeth, you will only remove it by visiting your dentist for a scale and polish.

2. Preventing tooth decay and cavities

One review of 12 studies found that people who brushed and flossed regularly were less likely to have bleeding gums. They had lower levels of gum inflammation (called gingivitis, the earliest stage of gum disease), too.

3. Preventing gum disease

By removing plaque from between your teeth and along/below the gum line where your tooth brushing cannot reach, you are reducing your chance of gum disease. Periodontal disease affects as many as half the number of adults, and while some people are more prone to it than others, it can affect anyone.

You definitely want to get the benefits that come from flossing. However, with floss possibly leading to bleeding gums, we also do NOT want to use floss that is made with the toxins we have discussed prior. So before you start flossing, or if you are already flossing and are going to continue, it is imperative that you look for nontoxic floss.

How to floss properly: a step-by-step guide

Here is a step-by-step guide to proper flossing. Of course, if you have any questions, you can always speak with your dentist or hygienist who will be happy to demo for you.

- Take about 16-20 inches of dental floss and wrap it around your middle fingers, leaving only about an inch or two of floss to work with.
- Holding the floss with your thumbs and index fingers, carefully guide the floss between your teeth, and in gentle sawing motion pop the floss between the tooth

contacts, being careful not to jam it into the gums.

- Once between the teeth, curve the floss into a C-shape, pressed tight against one tooth. Then, slide the floss up and down the tooth and root surface, going just under the gumline. Make sure to never force the floss further than it wants to go, since this action can irritate or lacerate your gum tissue. Repeat this process on the tooth on the other side of the space.

- To remove the floss, use the same back and forth sawing

motion to bring the floss up and away from the space between your teeth.

- Repeat this action for each tooth, using clean sections of floss as you move from space to space. Don't forget the back side of the last tooth in each corner of your mouth.

- Dispose of the dental floss in a trash can. It is important to never reuse a piece of floss as it will not be as effective, and could very much leave behind bacteria that you don't want in your mouth.

Brushing your teeth only reaches three out of five surfaces, so it's important to clean between them as well. The best way to do this is by flossing once a day. It is your choice which floss you would like to use, but I would only suggest staying away from any floss that may be made with toxic substances.

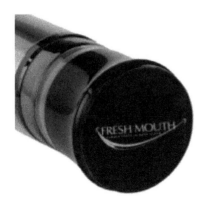

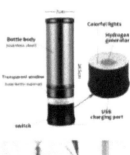

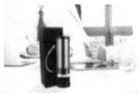

CHAPTER 7:

OZONE WATER

What is Ozone Water?

Ozone water is drinking water that has been purified through an ozone-based sterilization process. Ozone is like oxygen, O_2, except that it has an additional oxygen molecule making it O_3. It is an allotropic form of oxygen, and is an extremely powerful oxidizing agent. When ozone is dissolved in water it can be leveraged as a broad-spectrum biocide, destroying all cysts, viruses, bacteria, and other pathogens. It was first used in the treatment of commercially available water in 1904.

Ozone is created when electricity is discharged through an oxygen source. It is manufactured by modern ozone generators, which feature an oxygenated gas source that is then energized by a high voltage stream. This splits each O_2 molecule into a pair of common oxygen atoms. These recombine back into oxygen, O_2, and ozone, O_3.

BENEFITS FOR BODY AND BRAIN

Ozone is tasteless and doesn't change the taste of the water. Scientific studies prove that ozone kills many different bacteria and viruses. It has been proven effective against viruses such as E. coli, yeast, salmonella, listeria and many others.

Lack of water to the brain can cause numerous symptoms including problems with focus, memory, brain fatigue and brain fog, as well as headaches, sleep issues, anger, depression, and many more. Because the brain uses over 15% of all the oxygen in the body, Ozone is beneficial because it removes impurities and adds oxygen to the bloodstream, helping the brain function much more sufficiently and giving it a way to get more oxygen.

Ozonated Water makes it stronger and better able to fight infections.

Bearing in mind that Ozone has abilities to kill parasites and eliminate viruses, it makes sense that drinking cold ozonated water on an empty stomach regularly can detoxify your intestinal tract. Doing this has also been shown to fight Flu, burn fat, and kill certain bacteria.

ANTI-AGING

It seems like no matter what the problem might be or how long a doctor has gone to school, the best answer they can come up with for arthritis, diabetes, fatigue, stroke, cancer, impotence, overweight, constipation, digestive disorders, Alzheimer's, and every known medical condition is age. You would think that after all that schooling, all that experience, and all the supposed knowledge that one would be absolutely embarrassed to give such a scapegoat excuse like age, all because they don't have the brains or knowledge to actually pick up a book and find out. Instead of looking at the same medication they have prescribed that exacerbated the problem and seeing the damage it has done, they will instead defend the manufacturers of that product, which are the same people that the doctor listened to for "education" on the product.

We are in a time where there is not only more information at our fingertips than any of these medical schools could imagine, but there are also much more intelligent, safer, and healthier ways to handle diseases than the poison most doctors are prescribing. The information age that we are in not only gives us more information than most of these outdated dinosaurs, but it also gives us more information than Albert Einstein or Isaac Newton had at their disposal. I am not saying this makes me or anyone else smarter than the geniuses of the world, but I am saying that it allows us to look deeper into what might be causing certain ailments and the best way to reverse them or possibly eliminate them from coming back. Especially since the current method is not a cure or even medicine, but is simply just a temporary fix. Imagine if you had a razor that sliced open the skin on your arm. Naturally, most people would agree that putting a bandaid over it until it healed would be a great idea. What if that same blade was going to cut you again tomorrow, and the next day, and the day after that, and the following week, and months to come? Would this same band aid still be the best possible treatment? Even better, would you just continue to buy a new band aid each and every day for the rest of your life until finally the cut became so deep and so painful that death was just imminent?

I know that this sounds absurd to anyone that may be reading this, because obviously you would eliminate whatever it was that was cutting you open with the razor. Why is it that this is so obvious, but when it comes to eliminating what is causing our sicknesses, such as arthritis, diabetes, fatigue, stroke, cancer and the many others leading us to our death, we seem to think that we should just put that "band aid" over it each and everyday until it finally takes our life? Well, there are so many things out there that have been proven much better for us than the poison we have been lied to about. Here is one secret that we should all live by at this time: **IF THE MAINSTREAM TELLS YOU IT IS BAD OR THE POWERS THAT BE HAVE DEEMED SOMETHING UNSAFE, FIND THE INFORMATION FOR YOURSELF AND GET THE ANSWERS TO WHY.**

Chances are there was a reason, and it usually means that a very large company was going to lose billions of dollars. **DO NOT** use the most popular search engine, use a few different ones and you will see the varying information that you will find.

Ozone water is just one of the hundreds of things out there that can help you live a better, healthier life. If we pay close attention to some of the many benefits of ozone water, we can see how logically it can help in dozens of ways.

Here is a short list of different things that we can connect the dots to how one improvement can lead to another and so on. Improves…

1.   Circulation
2.   Energizes cells
3.   Enhances immune system
4.   Purifies skin

Ozone water therapy can help your circulation and energize your cells. If your body has better circulation with more enhanced energized cells, it will no doubt help to enhance and strengthen your immune system. With better circulation, energized cells and a stronger immune system, it would only make logical sense that your skin can be purer.

1.   Blood purifier

2.   Relieves muscle aches

3.   Burns fat

4.   Eliminates lactic acid

5.   Builds muscle

Strong blood circulation will help relieve muscle aches and soreness, so if that same blood is purer, even only a small percentage it is still going to help with muscle aches and pains to an even stronger degree in theory. If fat is being burned more efficiently, then it would make building muscle a lot easier, especially if you are doing the proper exercise regimen.

1. Neutralizes stomach acid
2. Kills parasites
3. Balances acid/alkaline
4. Improves mineral absorption and vitamin uptake
5. Kills some viruses and bacteria

PARASITES- A parasite is an organism that lives on or in a host and gets its food from or at the expense of its host.

A few other ways to describe a parasite would be words such as *freeloader, moocher, sponge, or leech.* These parasites depend on the host, which in our case would be us or the human body, for food and survival. So, imagine having another organism LIVING inside of YOU! Using YOUR body for food, warmth, and shelter. It almost sounds as if the parasite has become a part of you. Since they are actually alive inside of you, they do not want to kill you. A parasite wants to continue living just like you and me, however they do NOT shy away from causing diseases.

It has been estimated that more than 2 Billion people have been infected with a **brain parasite** spread by cat feces and contaminated meat, but most will never show symptoms. The University of Virginia researchers found that the parasite, **Toxoplasma gondii**, is kept in check by brain defenders called microglia. These microglia release a unique immune molecule, IL-1a, that recruits immune cells from the blood to control the parasite in the brain, the scientists discovered. This process works so well that very few people develop symptomatic toxoplasmosis, the disease the parasite causes. Many studies have shown that 85% of Americans have some sort of parasite, or 297 million people. Here is a list of symptoms you may see if you have a parasite.

Possible Parasite symptoms:

- Repeated diarrhea or constipation
- Chronic, unexplained nausea, often accompanied by vomiting
- Fatigue and weakness · Intestinal cramping
- Unexplained dizziness
- Foul-smelling flatulence

- Indigestion
- Bloating
- Multiple food allergies
- Loss of appetite
- Itching around the anus, especially at night
- Difficulty sleeping

- Difficulty maintaining a healthy weight (over or underweight)
- Itching on the soles of the feet, often accompanied by a rash
- Itching or tingling sensations on the scalp
- Coughing blood (severe cases)
- Palpitations (hookworms)
- Anemia
- Facial swelling around the eyes (roundworms)
- Wheezing and coughing, followed by vomiting, stomach pain and bloating (suggesting roundworms or threadworms)

We can go on and on about the different types of parasites, where they are from, and the countless scary things they can do. The point is, if 85% of people have parasites and these parasites survive by soaking up all the food, vitamins, minerals and nutrients you put in your mouth, it would only make sense that eliminating these parasites would help. By using Ozone water, it helps eliminate or at the very least decrease parasites, which help your body absorb vitamins, minerals and nutrients much more effectively.

Something else that would help with the absorption of vitamins and minerals would be neutralizing stomach acid and balancing acid/alkaline in the body. We can see why we would experience better mineral absorption, creating better vitamin uptake with Ozone water treatment. With all these benefits from Ozone water, we have a much stronger immune system now assisting in the elimination of viruses and bacteria. Other benefits include burning off excess sugar which can help with diabetes as well as better memory and improved brain function. The list goes on and on with the benefits of ozone water, however, another enormous benefit is for oral care. With an ozonized glass of water used as a type of mouthwash, or rinse, you can treat oral infections and kill the bad bacteria in your mouth. You can even take this a step further and combine this with the oil pulling we spoke about earlier. They have recently found that coconut oil and olive oil are great delivery systems for the ozone. So now you can do coconut oil pulling with ozone, making sure to fully eliminate as much bad bacteria as possible.

Dental ozone therapy is fast becoming one of the most effective treatment options used in dentistry today. Since our bodies have become so antibiotic-resistant, dentists have been turning to things such as silver and Ozone therapy. For oral care, Ozone can also clear away infections, as well as cavity-causing bacteria. Ozone can help reduce tooth sensitivity, and if used with a Nano-silver toothpaste the tooth sensitivity can be eliminated depending on the severity. It can also heal gum infections and support bone regeneration. Because of the anti-viral aspect it has been proven to eliminate canker sores quickly. Ozone is 1.5 times greater than chloride when used as an antimicrobial agent against bacteria, viruses, fungi, and protozoa, and because of this, it can also help disinfect areas of the mouth after a tooth extraction. This is something that should be an absolute must when getting a root canal to try and eliminate chances of infections.

Ozone

- Activation of aerobic processes (glycolysis, Krebs cycle). Seidler, 2008.
- Antimicrobial agent against bacteria, fungi, protozoa and viruses. Azarpazhood, Limeback (2008).
- Secretion of vasodilators (such as nitric oxide). Bocci, 2006; Seidler, 2008.
- Antioxidant capacity, enhance of the immune system, release of growth factors. Bocci 2006.
- Induces synthesis of interleukins and leukotrienes. Seidler (2008).
- Expression of adaptive inflammatory responses. Valacchi, Fortino, Bocci (2005).

Conclusion

It turns out that more women will make it a point to brush their teeth twice daily, while men tend to not be as serious about following a specific regimen or system. Men are also less likely to brush after each meal, leaving the food particles in between the teeth to rot.

To put things in perspective, 28.7% of women will brush after each meal, and 56.8% of them will brush twice a day, while 20.5% of men will brush after meals and 49% will brush twice daily.

Poor oral hygiene habits along with poor diet could increase the risk of problems developing. This could be the apparent reason why men are also more likely to exhibit decay that has been left untreated (29% of men compared to 25% of women between the ages of 35 and 44).

Research has found that 34% of men between 30-54 years of age already have gum disease/periodontal disease. This is inflammation of the gums that, if allowed to progress, can lead to the loss of the tissues that hold your teeth in place. I hope at this point you are seeing how bad this is, not just for your health, but how you look and carry yourself. This is compared to 23% of women in that age group. And it gets worse as men get older, as 56% of men between 55-90 years of age have periodontal disease, compared to 44% of women. If you happen to be one of those on the bottom end of these statistics, **PLEASE, PLEASE, PLEASE, START TAKING BETTER CARE OF YOUR TEETH!!!!!**

Here are a few ideas of the things that we can do to stop cavities, gum disease, halitosis, root canals and overall losing our teeth altogether.

- brush your teeth twice a day

- clean between your teeth with floss or another interdental cleaner once every day.
- Brush with all-natural toothpaste that has an antibacterial agent such as Nano-silver.
- Rinse with ozone water.
- If you use mouthwash, make sure it is alcohol-free.
- Disinfect your brush head.
  Use only soft bristles on your toothbrush.
  Change your brush every month to avoid fraying and bacteria entering your bloodstream.
- Try not to store your toothbrush in the bathroom, especially if you

share a bathroom with anyone else.

CPSIA information can be obtained
at www.ICGtesting.com
Printed in the USA
LVHW081534120522
718524LV00007B/334

9 781088 028166